FOOT AND ANKLE
PAIN

EDITION 2

FOOT AND ANKLE PAIN

RENE CAILLIET, M.D.

Professor and Chairman
Department of Rehabilitative Medicine
University of Southern California
School of Medicine
Los Angeles, California

Illustrations by R. Cailliet, M.D.

 F. A. DAVIS COMPANY • Philadelphia

Also by Rene Cailliet:

Low Back Pain Syndrome
Shoulder Pain
Neck and Arm Pain
Knee Pain and Disability
Soft Tissue Pain Disability
Hand Pain

Library of Congress Cataloging in Publication Data

Cailliet, Rene.
  Foot and ankle pain.

  Includes bibliographical references and index.
    1. Foot—Abnormalities.   2. Foot—Diseases.
3. Foot—Wounds and injuries.   I. Title.
RD781.C33   1983   617'.585   82-9967
ISBN 0-8036-1601-5   AACR2

Preface

Man's foot is subjected to daily stresses and strains. It is cramped into illfitting shoes, made to walk on hard surfaces, and allowed to become debilitated by constant trauma and misuse. The study of the bones and muscles of the foot during medical training is too often presented in an uninteresting and confusing manner with no correlation to function. Care of the ailing foot is then relegated to the unscientifically trained shoe salesman or boot maker.

The foot presents a segment of the human anatomy that is accessible to examination, palpation, and complete mechanical evaluation. No portion of the foot escapes the discerning eye if the functional anatomy is clearly understood.

The history given by the patient describes misuse of the foot, and the examination verifies the mechanism causing the pain. As in previous volumes of the Pain Series, the first portion of this book is devoted to normal functional anatomy. Subsequent chapters discuss various painful conditions and how each is related to the abnormal mechanism causing the pain and disability. Logical treatment that attempts to correct or alter the abnormality discovered from the history and physical examination is described.

New chapters in this edition include: The Foot in Running and Jogging, The Foot in Rhematoid Arthritis, and The Foot in Diabetes. The remaining chapters have been extensively updated and revised to include the latest information.

RENE CAILLIET, M.D.

Contents

Illustrations

CHAPTER 1

Structural Anatomy

The foot is a complex unit composed of twenty-six bones that can bear the full-body weight on standing and is able to transport the human body. The twenty-six bones consist of fourteen phalanges, five metatarsals, and seven tarsal bones. The foot can be divided into three functional segments (Fig. 1). (1) The posterior segment lies directly under the tibia and supports it. This segment contains the talus at the apex of the foot (part of the ankle joint) and the calcaneus (hind portion of the foot in contact with the ground). (2) The middle segment contains five tarsal bones that form an irregular rhomboid with medial base and lateral apex. The three cuneiforms and the anterior part of the cuboid form a row with the navicular bone and the posterior portion of the cuboid behind. (3) The anterior segment of the foot contains five metatarsal and fourteen phalangeal bones. The big toe has two phalanges, whereas the outer toes contain three each.

BONES AND LIGAMENTS

The foot can best be understood structurally and functionally if each bone is related in position and movement to the others. The *talus* is the mechanical keystone at the apex of the foot. It has a body, neck, and head. The superior surface and both sides of the body support and articulate with the tibia and fibula. The convex, saddle-shaped, superior surface of the talus glides under the tibia during ankle motion (Fig. 2).

The two sides and the superior surface of the talus are covered with articular cartilage and are "gripped" between the tibial and tibular malleoli that form the ankle mortise. The tibial malleolus extends about one third of the way down the medial surface of the body of the talus, whereas the fibular malleolus covers its entire lateral surface. The superior portion of the body supports the tibia. Within this mortise, the talus functions as a hinge joint.

1

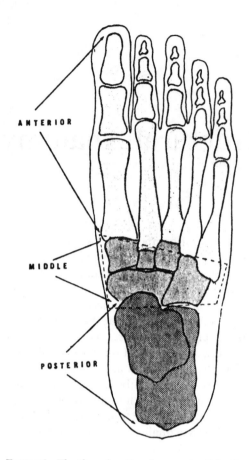

FIGURE 1. The three functional segments of the foot.

When viewed from above, the mortise is laterally angled since the medial malleolus is anterior to the lateral malleolus in the transverse plane (Fig. 3). The body of the talus is wedge-shaped with the wider portion anterior. As the ankle dorsiflexes (Fig. 4), this wider portion comes up between the two malleoli and wedges between them. Plantar flexion of the foot presents the posterior narrower portion of the talus between the malleoli and in this position permits some lateral motion of the talus within the mortise. This mobility creates instability of the joint and places an added burden on its supporting ligaments.

Ligaments provide further stability to the ankle joint. The integrity of the mortise is maintained by the interosseous ligament and membrane, and the anterior and posterior tibiofibular ligaments. The interosseous ligament attaches to the inner aspect of the tibia and proceeds laterally

2

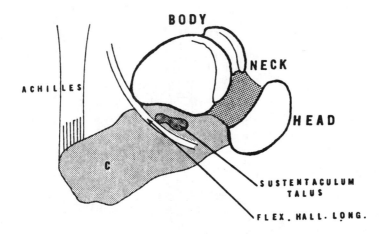

FIGURE 2. Talus. The talus is at the apex of the posterior segment of the foot. It is divisible into a body, neck, and head. The body has two articular surfaces that fit into the ankle mortise. The head articulates with the middle segment, and the entire talus fits upon and articulates with the calcaneus (C).

and downward to the inner aspect of the fibula. The fibula rises slightly during ankle dorsiflexion (Fig. 5) and causes the fibers to become more nearly horizontal, thus widening the mortise as the wider portion of the talus enters it. With full dorsiflexion, the mortise is fully expanded and further dorsiflexion is checked. Plantar flexion presents the narrower portion of the talus within the mortise, the fibula rides down, returning the interosseous ligament to its oblique course. The mortise here is narrower. The interosseous ligament and membrane are reinforced by the posterior and anterior tibiofibular ligaments that run parallel to the interosseous ligament. These ligaments may be torn in severe ankle sprains and fractures.

The ankle joint receives its strongest support from the collateral ligaments. The lateral collateral ligament supports the lateral aspect of the ankle and is composed of three bands: (1) the anterior talofibular ligament, which originates on the neck of the talus and attaches to the tip of the fibula, (2) the calcaneofibular ligament, which runs from the calcaneus to the tip of the fibula, and (3) the posterior talofibular ligament, which runs from the body of the talus to the tip of the fibula (Fig. 6).

The anterior talofibular and the calcaneofibular ligaments are the ones most frequently injured when the ankle is sprained. This is usually an inversion injury while the ankle is in its most unstable position (i.e., plantar flexion).

The medial aspect of the ankle joint is strongly supported by the deltoid ligament, which courses from the medial malleolus to the navicular, the

3

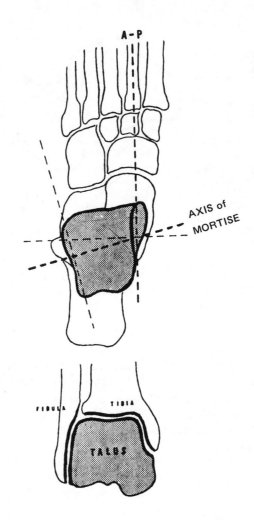

FIGURE 3. Superior view of the talus. Viewed from above the talus is wedge-shaped being wider anteriorly. It fits between the tibial and fibular malleoli that form the mortise.

sustentaculum talus, and the posterior aspect of the talus. The deltoid ligament is composed of four bands: (1) tibionavicular, (2) anterior talotibial, (3) calcaneotibial, and (4) posterior talotibial. The deltoid ligament is so strong that severe eversion stress upon the ankle will usually cause avulsion of the malleolus rather than a tear of this ligament.

Dorsiflexion and plantar flexion of the ankle occur about an axis that passes transversely through the body of the talus (see Figs. 3 and 4). The lateral end of the ankle axis passes through the tip of the fibula and is centrally located between the attachments of the lateral collateral liga-

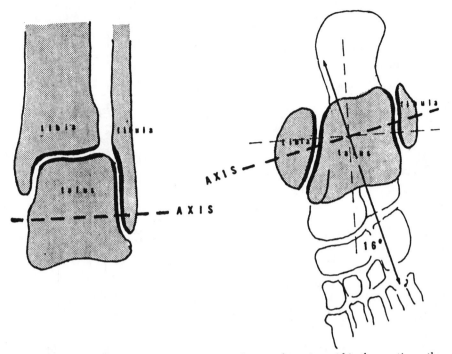

FIGURE 4. Ankle mortise and talus relationship. The axis of rotation within the mortise as the ankle plantar flexes and dorsiflexes is shown on the left. It passes through the fibula but below the tip of the tibia. Viewed from above, the tibia is anterior to the fibula forming an external "toe out" of 16°.

ments (Fig. 7), allowing them to remain taut during all movements. At its medial end, the transverse axis is placed eccentrically to the point of attachment of the medial ligaments. In this situation, the posterior medial ligaments become taut on dorsiflexion and the anterior medial ligaments become taut on plantar flexion. This arrangement of alternating tautness and slackness restricts the range of plantar and dorsal motion of the ankle.

The subtalar joint (talocalcaneal joint) contains several joints in different planes that permit simultaneous movements in different directions. The subtalar joint is divided into two synovia-lined chambers by an oblique canal formed by a groove in the talus and a corresponding groove in the calcaneus. The grooves, respectively termed the sulcus talus and the sulcus calcaneus, when opposed, form the tarsal canal. The canal is funnel-shaped with the wide portion at its lateral end. The lateral opening, the sinus tarsi, can be palpated in front of the fibular malleolus, especially when the foot is markedly inverted. The canal proceeds medially and posteriorly to its medial opening just behind and above the sustantaculum talus.

5

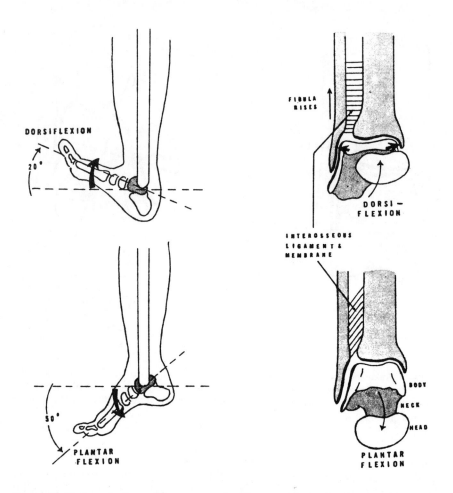

FIGURE 5. Motion of talus within mortise: dorsiflexion and plantar flexion. As the ankle dorsiflexes, the wider anterior portion of the talus wedges in the mortise and the fibula rises causing the interosseous ligament to become horizontal. When the mortise has been fully expanded, it prevents further dorsiflexion. On plantar flexion, the narrow portion of the talus presents itself and the fibula descends. Here the fibers resume their oblique direction and the mortise decreases its width.

The posterior facet of the subtalar joint (Fig. 8) is convex on the superior surface of the calcaneus and concave on the inferior surface of the talus. Motion at this joint is principally that of inversion and eversion (Fig. 9) with the calcaneus providing most of this motion as the talus is "locked" within the mortise. This motion can be tested clinically by first placing the foot in marked dorsiflexion, thus "locking" the talus, then grasping the calcaneus to elicit lateral and medial motion.

6

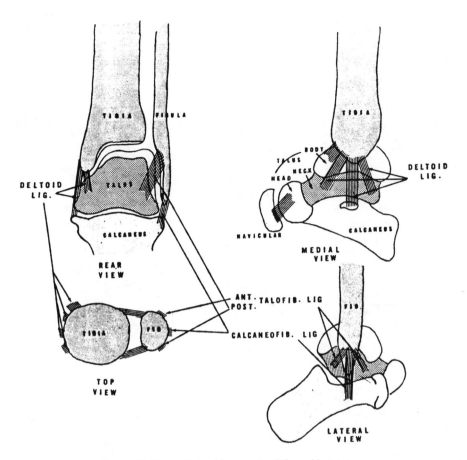

FIGURE 6. The collateral ligaments of the ankle joint.

The anterior and middle facets of the subtalar joint (see Fig. 8) consist of two similar surfaces on the superior aspect of the calcaneus and the inferior aspect of the body and neck of the talus. The facets of the neck and body of the talus are convex, and those of the calcaneus are concave. This is exactly contrary to the relationship of the posterior facet of the subtalar joint in which the calcaneal facet is convex and the talar facet of the joint is concave.

The talonavicular joint is related to the subtalar joint and is formed by the fitting of the large convex surface of the head of the talus into the posterior concave surface of the navicular bone (Fig. 10). This joint is a part of the transverse tarsal joint.

The subtalar axis about which the calcaneus rotates in respect to the talus has a 45° angle to the floor and a 16° angle medial to a line drawn

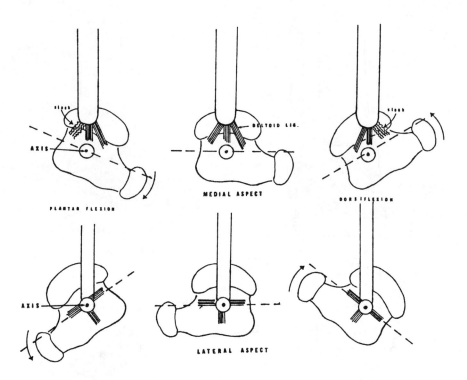

FIGURE 7. Relationship of medial and lateral collateral ligaments to the axis of ankle motion. The transverse axis of the mortise transects the center of attachment of the lateral ligaments at the tip of the fibula. Plantar flexion or dorsiflexion of the ankle does not change the length of the ligaments. The axis is eccentric to the medial deltoid ligament. During plantar flexion, the posterior strands become slack and the anterior fibers taut. The opposite occurs during dorsiflexion.

through the second metatarsal (Fig. 11). Three types of movement occur in combination about this axis: (1) *inversion,* which consists of elevation of the medial border and depression of the lateral border of the foot about the longitudinal axis, and the opposite movement of *eversion,* (2) *abduction,* which is outward rotation about a vertical axis through the tibia, and *adduction,* which is inward rotation, and (3) *dorsiflexion* and *plantar flexion* about the transverse axis. This last type of movement is similar to but significantly less than the motion of the talus on the tibia.

When all of these types of subtalar motions occur simultaneously, they result in *supination* of the foot, a combination of inversion, adduction, and plantar flexion, or *pronation* of the foot, a combination of eversion, abduction, and dorsiflexion.

The interosseous talocalcaneal ligament (see Fig. 8) binds the calcaneus to the talus. It runs the length of the tarsal canal and forms a partition

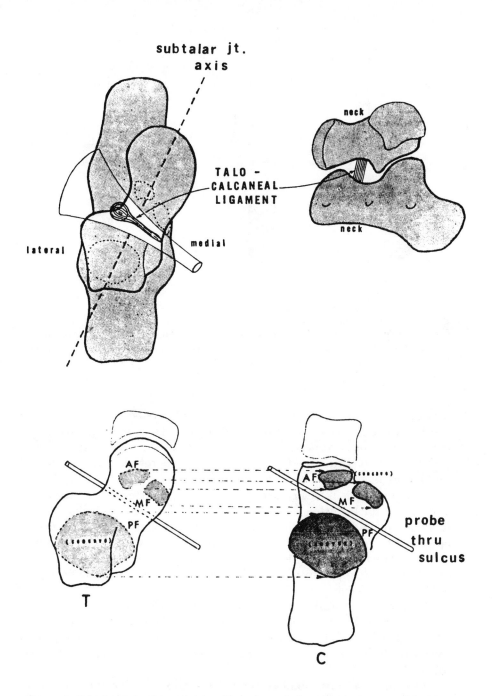

FIGURE 8. Subtalar (talocalcaneal) joint. The talus and the calcaneus are joined by three facets. anterior (AF), middle (MF), and posterior (PF). The sinus tarsi (tarsal canal) in its oblique course contains the talocalcaneal ligament that binds the two bones.

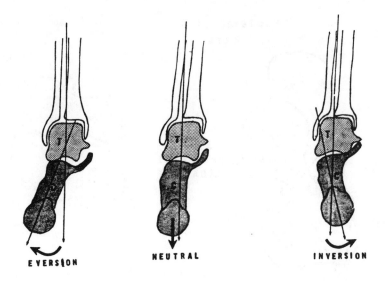

FIGURE 9. Motion of the subtalar (talocalcaneal) joint. The talus is fixed within the mortise and has no lateral motion. The calcaneus has medial and lateral motion upon the inferior surface of the talus. The degree of inversion and eversion is restricted by the talocalcaneal ligament and the collateral ligaments of the ankle.

between the anterior and posterior portions of the talocalcaneal joints. At its fibular end there is a discrete fibrous band (ligamentum cervicis) that connects two small tubercles opposing each other on the talus and the calcaneus. This firm band, about which some rotation can occur, is termed the ligamentum cervicis.

The interosseous talocalcaneal ligament tenses during inversion of the foot and is slack during eversion because it runs perpendicular to the subtalar axis and most of the ligament plus the ligamentum cervicis lies lateral to it. This ligamentous action increases the stability of the supinated foot. The interosseous ligament can be palpated at the large opening of the tarsal canal just in front of the fibular malleolus when the canal is opened by inversion.

The degree of inversion or eversion of the subtalar joint is further limited by a small bony process located on the lateral inferior aspect of the body of the talus that impinges upon a similar process on the adjacent calcaneus. These processes contact upon eversion of the heel and restrict further eversion.

The transverse tarsal joint consists of the talonavicular and the calcaneocuboid joints. It has been termed the "surgeon's tarsal joint," the midtarsal joint, or Chopart's joint and is often the site of amputation of the foot.

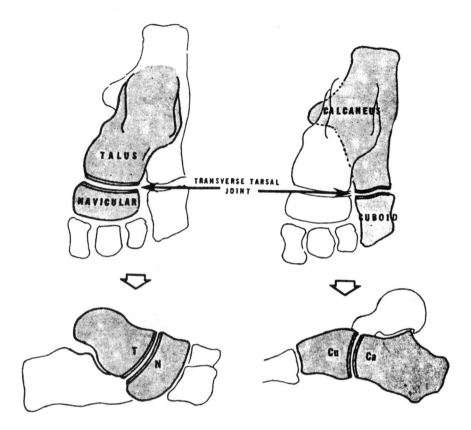

FIGURE 10. Transverse tarsal joint.

The rounded head of the talus fits into the cupped surface of the navicular. Motion of this joint is that of rotation about an axis through the talus, which slants in a forward, downward, and medial direction. The articular surface of the head of the talus is larger than the adjoining surface of the navicular, which permits significant gliding at the talonavicular joint allowing inversion and eversion of the foot.

The calcaneocuboid joint has a limited range of motion permitting some abduction and adduction. When the axis of the talonavicular joint runs parallel to the axis of the calcaneocuboid joint, total motion is free and the foot is unstable. This is the situation in the pronated foot. When the two axes diverge, as in the supinated foot, motion of the transverse tarsal joint is restricted and the foot is more stable. This function plus the tautness of the interosseous ligament are the reasons for the foot being most stable in the supinated position.

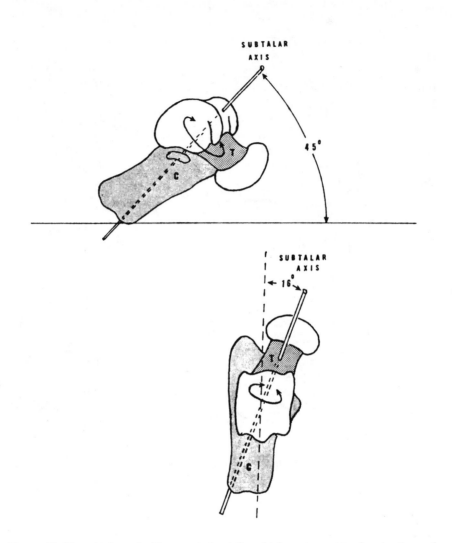

FIGURE 11. The subtalar axis. Movement about the subtalar axis consists of supination and pronation of the foot. The axis forms a 45° angle with the ground and a 16° angle medial to a longitudinal line drawn through the second metatarsal.

The tarsal joints distal to the subtalar joint produce the elasticity of the foot that permits accommodation to uneven surfaces when walking. However, the modern, firm, inflexible shoe markedly restricts this motion.

The middle functional segment (see Fig. 1) consists of five tarsal bones: the navicular, the cuboid, and the three cuneiforms. A rigid transverse arch held together by the interosseous ligaments is formed by the cuneiform bones and the cuboid, the middle cuneiform being the keystone (Fig. 12).

The anterior margin of the middle segment does not present a straight border to the bases of the metatarsal bones. The second cuneiform is set back forming an indentation into which the base of the second metatarsal is formly wedged. Being situated between the first and third cuneiforms, the second metatarsal moves only in plantar flexion and dorsiflexion, articulating at its base with the first and third cuneiforms.

The bases of the third, fourth, and fifth metatarsals are obliquely shaped, permitting a rotatory motion of the third upon the second, the

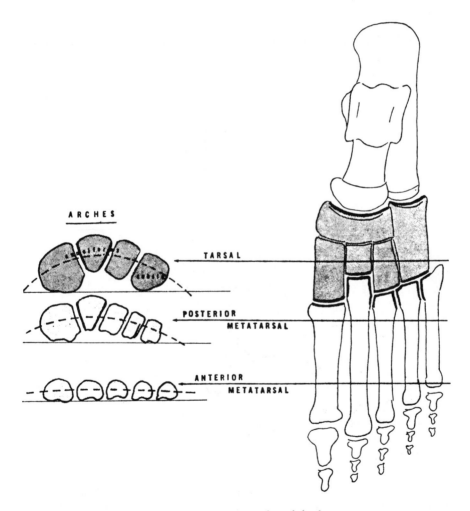

FIGURE 12. The transverse arches of the foot.

13

fourth upon the third, and the fifth around the fourth. The fifth metatarsal, contacting only the base of the fourth and the cuboid, moves through the greatest arc. This rotatory motion increases the transverse arch and thus "cups" the sole of the foot. The base of the fifth metatarsal protrudes laterally to form a sulcus through which runs the tendon of the peroneus longus muscle.

The first metatarsal is the thickest and the shortest. It has a kidney-shaped base that permits not only dorsal and plantar flexion but also rotation about an arc around the base of the second metatarsal. The base is also shaped to permit gliding motion upon the surface of the first cuneiform. The anterior tibial and peroneus longus tendons attach upon the plantar surface of the first metatarsal (Fig. 13).

Under the head of the first metatarsal there are two small facets for the articulation of the two sesamoid bones. These sesamoid bones, erroneously called "accessory" bones, are incorporated into the tendons of the

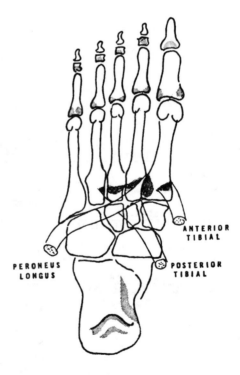

FIGURE 13. Tendons that attach to the base of the first metatarsal. Viewed from the plantar surface, the anterior tibial tendon attaches to the medial aspect and the peroneus longus tendon to the lateral aspect of the base of the first metatarsal.

flexor hallucis brevis and act as a fulcrum in the function of the tendon. They also bear body weight.

The forward projected length of the metatarsals follows a sequence of 2 > 3 > 1 > 4 > 5. The second metatarsal head protrudes the farthest, with the first metatarsal being shorter than the third (Fig. 14). Excessive shortening of the first metatarsal may have pathologic significance as it causes the second metatarsal head to bear excessive weight.

The phalanges articulate in a gliding manner upon the large convex articular surfaces of the metatarsal heads. These surfaces extend from the plantar surface of the metatarsal heads onto the dorsum of the heads, thus permitting excessive dorsiflexion of the toes. There are two phalanges in

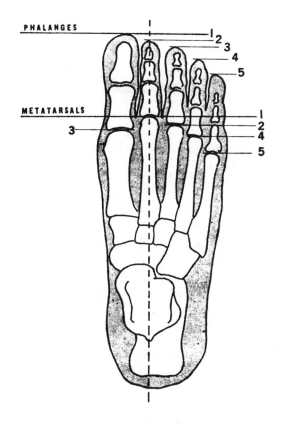

FIGURE 14. Relative length of projection of the metatarsals and the phalanges. The relative anterior protrusion of the metatarsals follows the pattern of 2 > 3 > 1 > 4 > 5. This makes the second metatarsal the longest and the first metatarsal the third longest. The toes have a pattern of 1 > 2 > 3 > 4 > 5 in which the first toe protrudes farthest forward followed by each adjacent toe in regular sequence.

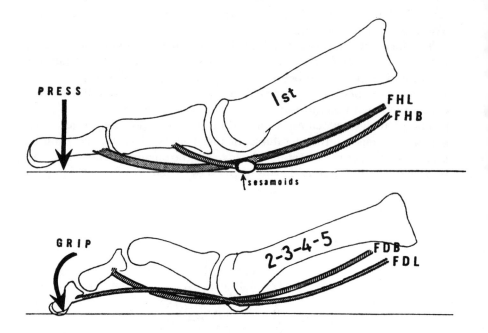

FIGURE 15. Action of the flexor tendons. The tendons of the big toe cross two joints and thus act by "pressing" the distal phalanx to the floor. The sesamoid bones are incorporated into the tendons of the flexor hallucis brevis (FHB) and act as a fulcrum for flexor action. The flexor tendons of the other toes cross three joints and act to "grip" the floor. This action is performed by the flexor digitorum brevis (FDB) and longus (FDL).

the first toe (hallux) and three in all the other toes. For proper range of motion, they should be in straight alignment and the capsules and tendons sufficiently flexible to allow full flexion and extension. In every step of walking, the big toe dorsiflexes; in a mile it dorsiflexes approximately 900 times. Improper alignment or lack of flexibility can traumatize the hallux joint.

Contrary to the relative forward projection of the metatarsal bones (2 > 3 > 1 > 4 > 5), the phalanges follow a sequence of 1 > 2 > 3 > 4 > 5. The first toe projects the farthest forward, with the other toes gradually decreasing (see Fig. 14).

The tendinous action upon the phalanges of the first toe differs from all the others. Because the big toe has only two phalanges, flexor action causes the distal phalanx to "press" against the ground. There is little proximal flexion (Fig. 15). Since the other four toes each have three phalanges, the tendons cross three joints causing a "gripping" action of the toes.

16

MUSCLES

Muscles that originate* away from the foot and act upon the foot constitute the *extrinsic* foot muscles (Fig. 16), whereas the *intrinsic* foot muscles originate and insert within the foot itself (Figs. 17 to 20).

The plantar flexors of the ankle are the powerful gastrocnemius and soleus muscles. The *gastrocnemius* originates above the knee by two heads, one connected to each femoral condyle. Halfway down the leg it ends in a flat tendon, the Achilles tendon, that attaches to the posterior aspect of the calcaneus and functions to plantar flex the ankle. When the foot is weight-bearing, the Achilles tendon elevates the heel from the floor. Due to the obliquity of the subtalar axis (see Fig. 11), the gastrocsoleus group is also a powerful spinator at the subtalar joint when the forefoot is fixed on the floor.

The *soleus* lies under the gastrocnemius and originates from the upper tibia and fibula below the knee joint. It acts upon the ankle joint but does not have ability to flex the knee as does the gastrocnemius. It ends as the deep portion of the Achilles tendon midway down the leg. With the foot fixed on the ground, the action of the gastroc-soleus group moves the tibia backward, a reversed origin-insertion action. With the knee flexed, the soleus is able to plantar flex the foot and ankle, whereas in the knee flexed position, the gastrocnemius loses its effectiveness.

During standing balance, with both feet planted firmly on the ground, lateral stability is maintained easily and muscular action is needed only to prevent forward and backward sway over the center of gravity. In the average stance, the feet evert to form an angle of 30°, and a plumb line dropped from the sacral promontory falls midway between the feet onto a line between the navicular bones (see Fig. 17). The long digital flexors (see Fig. 15) create a firm pressure of the toes on the ground, and the tendons that run down the medial side of the ankle afford lateral stability by preventing eversion of the anke.

In a relaxed stance, the plumb line passes 3° in front of the talus, and the gastroc-soleus group pulls the leg back to maintain balance (see Fig. 18). In relaxed erect stance, no muscular action is needed anywhere in the body other than the tonic contraction of the gastroc-soleus group. The

---

*The terms "origin" and "insertion" are used by most textbooks to describe muscular action with the distal appendage being free to move as the tendon and muscle direct. This description is far from accurate. During the "stance" phase of gait which constitutes 60 percent of the walking cycle, as well as during standing, the foot is fixed to the floor causing muscular action to act upon the proximal bones. The foot is now the "origin," and the attachment of the muscles to the lower leg now becomes the "insertion," a reversal of the ordinary textbook designation. The opposite occurs when the foot is non-weight bearing and thus a free-moving appendage. This dual role of muscular action is discussed further under Gait Determinants in Chapter 3.

17

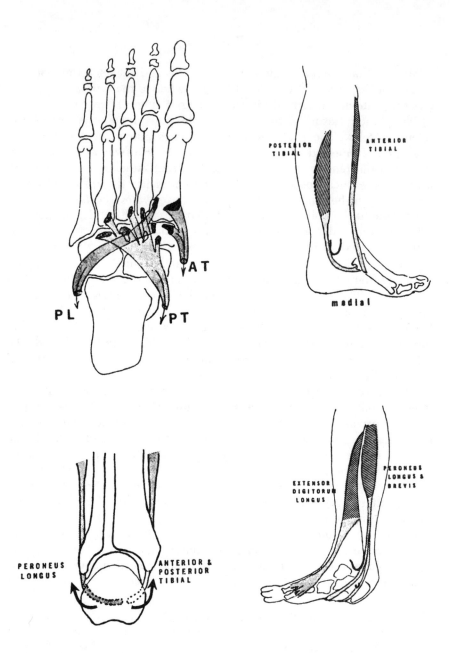

FIGURE 16. Extrinsic musculature of the foot. The origin, direction, and insertion of the extrinsic muscles acting upon the foot are shown. The anterior tibial (AT) and the posterior tibial (PT) are medial muscles that invert the foot. The peroneus longus (PL) everts the foot. Both the posterior tibial and the peroneus longus also plantar flex the foot. The extensor digitorum and the anterior tibial dorsiflex the foot.

18

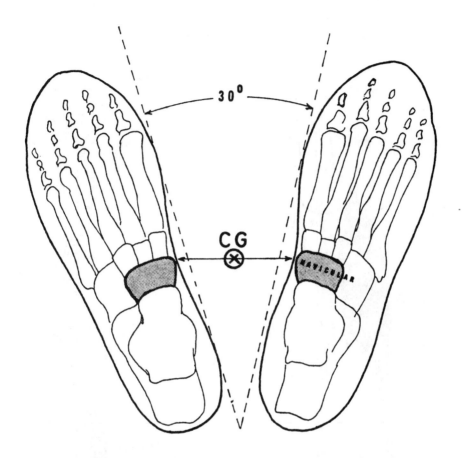

FIGURE 17. Center of gravity in two-legged stance. With the person standing and balancing on both feet, the feet describe an arc with the feet "toeing out" 30°. The center of gravity (CG) of the body is midway between the two navicular bones.

remainder of the support is ligamentous. Should the center of gravity shift posteriorly, the anterior leg muscles and the ankle dorsiflexors, with the foot fixed on the ground, pull the leg forward.

All the tendons passing behind the malleoli are considered plantar flexors. Medially, these are the tibialis posterior, the flexor digitorum longus, and the flexor hallucis longus. Laterally, the muscles consist of the peroneus longus and brevis. These groups of muscles contribute only 5 percent of the total pull used to lift the heel off the ground. The major responsibility for this action belongs to the gastroc-soleus muscles.

When stance is attempted on one foot, stability is dependent upon the lateral and medial tendons acting across the ankle joint. With the foot

19

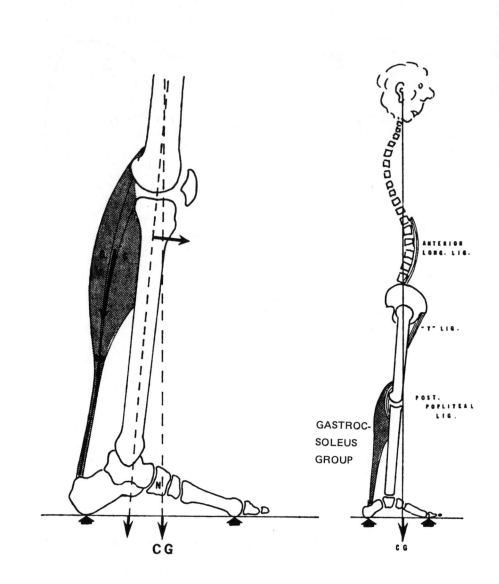

GASTROC-
SOLEUS
GROUP

ANTERIOR
LONG. LIG.

"Y" LIG.

POST.
POPLITEAL
LIG.

CG

CG

FIGURE 18. Muscular effort of relaxed two-legged standing position. In standing on both feet in a relaxed manner, the spine leans on the anterior longitudinal ligament, the hip on the iliofemoral (Y) ligament, and the knees extend to lean on the posterior popliteal ligaments. The gastroc-soleus must maintain tonus to pull the leg back because the center of gravity falls some 3° ahead of the talus. Relaxed erect posture is principally ligamentous with only the gastroc-soleus group active. (From Cailliet, R.: Low Back Pain Syndrome, ed. 3. F.A. Davis, 1968, with permission.)

fixed on the floor, the tendons crossing the medial half of the foot pull the leg medially and those crossing the lateral half pull laterally (see Fig. 16).

If the center of gravity shifts laterally to the talus during one-legged balance, the tendons on the medial aspect of the foot pull the leg medially over the foot. These muscles are principally the *tibialis posterior* and the *tibialis anterior* (see Fig. 19). This balancing adjustment requires very little muscular action. The sensory feedback from the plantar nerves initiates this coordinated muscular effort in both the specific muscle and the exact amount of contraction. Much of the sensory feedback comes from the toes that are forced to the ground, the big toe pressing and the other toes gripping (see Fig. 15). The muscular action involved in standing balance does not apply to muscular action when walking. This is discussed in Chapter 3.

The remainder of the lower leg muscles acting upon the foot are divided into three groups: lateral, anterior, and medial. The lateral group contains the *peroneus longus* and *brevis* arising from the lateral aspect of

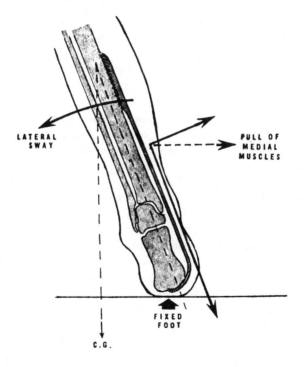

FIGURE 19. Muscular action for lateral stability in one-legged stance. As the body sways lateral to the center of gravity (CG), the medial muscles (tibialis anterior and tibialis posterior) act from the fixed foot to pull medially.

21

the fibula. The longus arises higher upon the fibula and is the most superficial. Both of their tendons share a common synovial sheath as they pass behind the lateral malleolus. The peroneus brevis attaches to the base of the fifth metatarsal while the peroneus longus runs deeply across the plantar surface of the foot and attaches to the base of the first metatarsal and the medial cuneiform (see Fig. 13). Their primary function is to evert the ankle.

The anterior group of muscles is comprised of the extensor digitorum longus, peroneus tertius, extensor hallucis longus, and tibialis anterior. The *tibialis anterior* originates from the lateral aspect of the tibia, crosses the dorsum of the foot, and inserts upon the medial cuneiform and the base of the first metatarsal (see Fig. 13). Its action is that of inversion and dorsiflexion of the foot. The *extensor hallucis longus* arises from the anterior surface of the fibula and the interosseous membrane, passes across the dorsum of the foot, and inserts upon the distal phalanx of the great toe. Its action is that of extension of the hallux. It also assists to dorsiflex the ankle. The *extensor digitorum longus* originates from the lateral condyle of the tibia and the anterior surface of the fibula and attaches by way of four tendons into the dorsal aspects of the four lateral toes. Each tendon divides at its end into a central slip that inserts upon the middle phalanx, and two slips that divide and insert upon the distal phalanx. The *peroneus tertius* seems to be part of the extensor digitorum longus but attaches to the base of the fifth metatarsal bone. The extensor digitorum longus extends the toes and together with the peroneus tertius assists in dorsiflexion and eversion of the foot.

The medial group of lower leg muscles contains the tibialis posterior, flexor digitorum longus, and flexor hallucis longus. Their tendons pass behind and under the medial malleolus. The *tibialis posterior* arises from the tibia and the fibula posteriorly and attaches by multiple fibrous extensions into most of the tarsals and medial metatarsals. Its function is inversion and plantar flexion of the foot. The *flexor hallucis longus* originates somewhat laterally from the fibula and the tibia and, from this posterior origin, passes obliquely across the lower leg to pass under the medial malleolus and attach upon the distal phalanx of the big toe. It crosses two joints and primarily acts to press the distal phalanx to the floor (see Fig. 15). The *flexor digitorum longus* arises from the posterior aspect of the tibia, passes behind the medial malleolus into the sole of the foot, and attaches to the distal phalanx of the four lateral toes. Its action is flexion of the toes in a "gripping" manner.

Inversion of the foot takes place at the subtalar and the transverse tarsal joints by means of tendons that traverse the inner border of the foot. Eversion occurs also at the subtalar joints by action of the laterally placed tendons. The peronei act most effectively as evertors when the foot is plantar flexed, and though they are mechanically situated to plantar flex

22

the foot, they do so ineffectively. Both evertors and inventors of the ankle act as stabilizers when the foot is fixed on the floor.

The muscles of the sole of the foot, commonly called the *intrinsics* of the foot, cannot be tested individually with any clinical significance. Their major function is that of "cupping" the sole of the foot, and their innervation is from the medial and lateral plantar branches of the posterior tibial nerve. They function vitally as a source of strength to the natural longitudinal arch of the foot in conjunction with the bony architecture of the foot, the ligamentous stability, and the long muscles and their tendons that pass under the foot.

The muscles supplied by the medial plantar nerve (*abductor hallucis, flexor digitorum brevis, flexor hallucis brevis,* and the *first lumbrical*) function primarily to plantar flex the toes, especially the metatarsophalangeal joint of the big toe. They also stabilize the first toe phalanges at the final push-off during walking. The muscles supplied by the lateral plantar nerve maintain the arches of the foot, flex the remaining toes at the metatarsophalangeal joints, and adduct and abduct the toes. This last function is lost in many people, but the major function discernible clinically is the power of flexion at the metatarsophalangeal joints. Detailed anatomic discussion of the muscles of the sole of the foot is intentionally omitted and the reader is referred to textbooks in anatomy. The four layers of muscle are shown in Figures 20 to 23, and the specific innervation is summarized in Figure 24.

The *plantar fascia* is a continuation of the plantaris tendon. Its origin is upon the medial tubercle of the calcaneus from which it proceeds anteri-

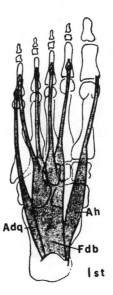

FIGURE 20. Muscles of the sole of the foot: first layer.
Adq = Abductor digiti quinti
Ah = Abductor hallucis
Fdb = Flexor digitorum brevis

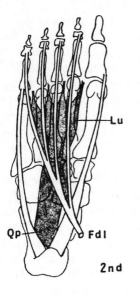

FIGURE 21. Muscles of the sole of the foot: second layer.
Qp = Quadratus plantae
Lu = Lumbricales
Fdl = Tendon of flexor digitorum longus

orly and splits into five bands to attach to each digit. Each band splits at the metatarsophalangeal joint to attach to the inner and outer sides of the joints and their plantar ligaments (Fig. 25). Through this split in the plantar fascia pass the long and short flexor tendons.

The medial and lateral portions of the fascia cover the abductors and short flexors of the big and little toes. There is frequently a short fibrous

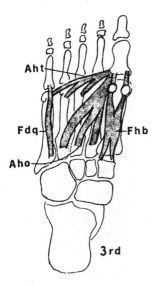

FIGURE 22. Muscles of the sole of the foot: third layer.
Aht = Adductor hallucis: transverse head
Aho = Adductor hallucis: oblique head
Fhb = Flexor hallucis brevis
Fdq = Flexor digiti quinti brevis

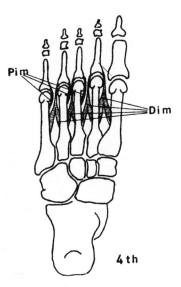

FIGURE 23. Muscles of the sole of the foot: fourth layer.
Pim = Plantar interosseous muscles
Dim = Dorsal interosseous muscles

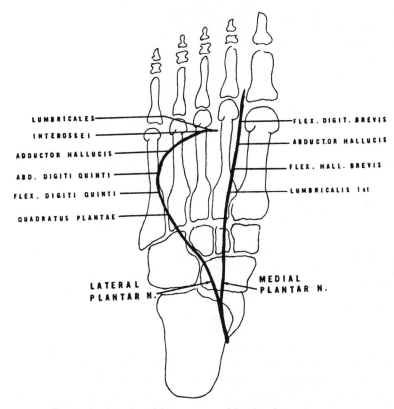

FIGURE 24. Muscles of foot innervated by the plantar nerves.

25

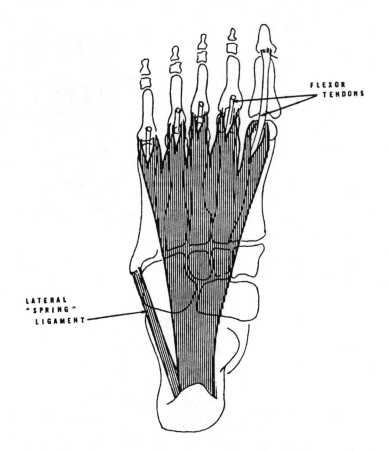

FLEXOR
TENDONS

LATERAL
"SPRING"
LIGAMENT

FIGURE 25. Plantar fascia. The plantar fascia originates from the calcaneal tubercle. Anteriorly it splits at each metatarsophalangeal joint to permit passage of the flexor tendons. A fibrous lateral band proceeds forward to attach to the base of the fifth metatarsal which forms part of the lateral "spring" ligament.

band that projects from the lateral aspect of the calcaneal tubercle to attach to the base of the fifth metatarsal and forms part of the lateral spring of the longitudinal arch.

NERVE SUPPLY

The nerves to the muscles of the lower leg and foot are shown in Figure 26. The *sciatic nerve* ends at the upper angle of the popliteal space where it divides into the tibial and the common peroneal nerves.

The *tibial nerve* is essentially a continuation of the sciatic nerve and enters the lower leg between the two heads of the gastrocnemius and

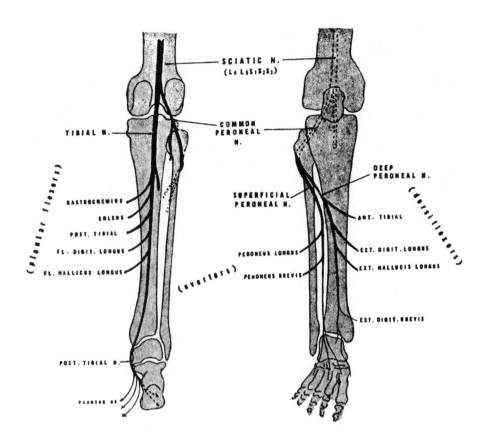

FIGURE 26. Innervation of the leg and foot. The sciatic nerve divides at the popliteal angle to form the tibial nerve and the common peroneal nerve.

passes deep to the soleus to enter the posterior compartment of the leg. It terminates in divisions of the plantar nerves, a medial and lateral plantar branch (see Fig. 26). The tibial nerve supplies the posterior muscles of the leg and innervates the plantar flexors of the foot.

The *medial plantar nerve* sends cutaneous sensory branches to the plantar surface of the medial three toes and the medial aspect of the fourth toe. Its motor branches supply the abductor hallucis, flexor hallucis brevis, flexor digitorum brevis, and the first two lumbricales (see Figs. 21 to 24).

The *lateral plantar nerve* passes across the plantar surface of the foot and, after dividing into deep and superficial branches, supplies the sensation to the plantar surface of the remaining toes on the lateral aspect of the foot. It supplies the motor innervation to the quadratus plantae,

27

flexor digiti quinti brevis, abductor digiti quinti, and the remaining plantar interosseous and lumbrical muscles.

The other division of the sciatic nerve, the *common peroneal nerve*, passes laterally out of the popliteal space, behind the head of the fibula beneath the deep fascia, and winds around the lateral aspect of the fibular neck. The common peroneal nerve supplies no musculature. It merely supplies small nerve twigs to the knee joint and ultimately divides into the superficial and deep peroneal nerves (see Fig. 26). The superficial peroneal nerve descends the leg in front of the fibula and supplies the evertor muscles of the foot. The sensory area of the superficial peroneal nerve is the lateral aspect of the lower leg and the dorsum of the foot. The deep peroneal nerve proceeds to the interosseous membrane between the tibia and fibula, and descends the leg supplying the dorsiflexors of the foot and ends supplying the extensor digitorum brevis. It supplies a small area of sensation between the first two toes on the dorsum of the foot. Both the deep and the superficial peroneal nerves terminate in sensory branches that supply the dorsum of the foot and anterolateral aspect of the leg (Fig. 27).

BLOOD SUPPLY

The *popliteal artery* is a direct continuation of the femoral artery that passes into the posterior popliteal quadrant and divides into the anterior

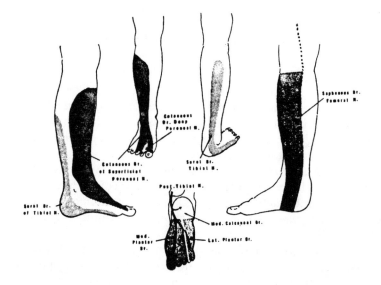

FIGURE 27. Sensory patterns of peripheral nerves of the leg.

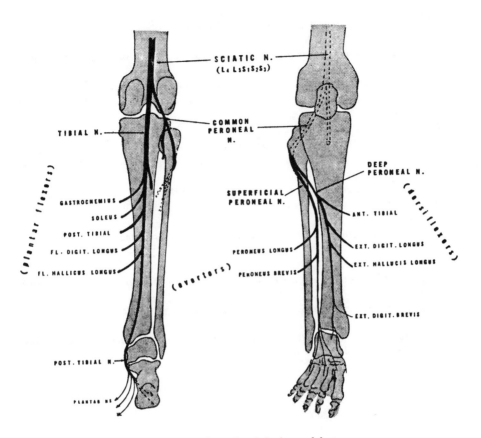

FIGURE 28. Arterial supply of the leg and foot.

and posterior tibial arteries going below the knee (Fig. 28). The *posterior tibial artery* follows the same course as the tibial nerve (see Fig. 26) and supplies the posterior muscles of the leg. Upon reaching the medial malleolus, it passes to the plantar surface of the foot to divide into the medial and lateral plantar arteries. Below the bifurcation, the *posterior tibial artery* branches off laterally into the *peroneal artery*, passes across the interosseous membrane, and descends the lateral aspect of the leg to supply the lateral muscles. It ends as the *lateral calcaneal artery*.

The *anterior tibial artery* passes anteriorly between the tibia and fibula, across the upper margin of the interosseous membrane, and then courses down the anterior surface of the membrane. It supplies the muscles of the anterior compartment of the leg and reaches the dorsum of the foot as the *dorsalis pedis artery*. The terminal branches form the *dorsal metatarsal arteries* and *dorsal digital arteries*, and communicate with the plantar distal branches of the plantar arteries.

BIBLIOGRAPHY

GOSS, CM (ED): *Gray's Anatomy of the Human Body,* ed 29. Lea & Febiger, Philadelphia, 1973.

GRANT, JC BOILEAU: *A Method of Anatomy,* ed 5. Williams & Wilkins, Baltimore, 1952.

HAYMAKER, W AND WOODHALL, B: *Peripheral Nerve Injuries: Principles of Diagnosis,* ed 2. WB Saunders, Philadelphia, 1959.

HICKS, JH: *Axis rotation at ankle joint.* J Anat 86:1. 1952.

HICKS, JH: *Mechanics of the foot.* J Anat 87:345, 1953.

HOLLINSHEAD, WH AND JENKINS, DB: *Functional Anatomy of the Limbs and Back,* ed 5. WB Saunders, Philadelphia, 1981.

JONES, FW: *Talocalcaneal articulation.* Lancet 2:241, 1944.

JONES, FW: *Structures and Function as Seen in the Foot,* ed 2. Bailliere, Tindall, and Cox, London, 1949.

KAPLAN, E: *Some principles of anatomy and kinesiology in stabilizing operations of the foot.* Clin Orthop 34:7, 1964.

LAKE, NC: *The Foot,* ed 3. Bailliere, Tindall, and Cox, London, 1943.

LAPIDUS, PW: Kinesiology and mechanical anatomy of the tarsal joints. Clin Orthop 30:20, 1963.

MENNELL, J: *The Science and Art of Joint Manipulation,* ed 2. J & A Churchill, London, 1949.

RUBIN, G AND WITTEN, M: *The talar tilt angle and the fibular collateral ligament.* J Bone Joint Surg 42A:311, March 1960.

CHAPTER 2

Examination of the Foot

The foot is one of the few segments of human anatomy that can be fully examined. All the significant functional elements of the foot are readily accessible, either visually, by palpation, or by passive motion by the examiner.

Pain, difficulty in walking, and awkwardness of gait are the foot problems that usually cause the patient to consult a physician. Foot pain may occur while standing or walking. The former may be considered the *static* foot and the latter the *kinetic*. Therefore, the foot must be examined during relaxation, weight bearing, and walking. The examiner must develop a meaningful pattern and sequence of examination to determine the cause of pain or dysfunction. Each of the criteria of the *normal foot* must be individually sought, and any·deviation from normal and its significance must be recognized and appreciated.

The *normal foot* conforms to the following criteria: (1) free of pain, (2) normal muscle balance, (3) absence of contracture, (4) a central heel, (5) straight and mobile toes, and (6) three sites of weight bearing while standing and during the stance phase of walking.

HISTORY

The first criterion is subjective and is revealed by the patient's history. The remaining criteria are objective and are elicited by the examination. If pain is the presenting complaint, the patient indicates the site of pain and relates its occurrence to a certain position, motion, or activity. The site of pain denotes the anatomic site of the disorder, and the examination reveals the cause.

If the complaint is an awkward, fatiguing, or cosmetically unpleasant gait, an exact description of the gait is elicited from the patient or companion. The examiner then witnesses and interprets the gait in question.

31

EXAMINATION OF THE SHOE

The patient's shoes are also examined as deformities of the heel, sole, or body of the shoe have diagnostic significance. The normal foot with normal gait should wear down the heel on its outer side. This generally indicates that the calcaneus is in the neutral position with the heel centrally placed and the foot slightly inverted, and also implies a good heel-toe gait. The everted foot distorts the counter (Fig. 29) and the quarter, and wears the heel on its inner border. A "drop foot" due to muscular weakness scuffs the toe of the shoe. The equinovarus of spastic paralysis may also cause abnormal wear of the shoe at the toe and outer border of the sole.

The deformed vamp may reveal anatomic abnormalities of the foot. Distortions here may be caused by tightness over hammer toes or hallux valgus with bunion formation. The worn areas of the sole indicate the position of the metatarsal heads (Fig. 30).

RANGE OF MOTION

Ankle

The major ranges of motion are tested during the examination of the bare foot. Ankle plantar flexion and dorsiflexion are tested both with the knee straight and with the knee bent. When the knee is straight, the

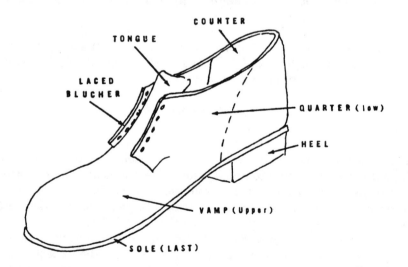

FIGURE 29. Components of the shoe.

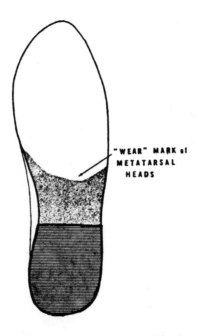

"WEAR" MARK of
METATARSAL
HEADS

FIGURE 30. Examination of the sole of the shoe.

gastrocnemius muscle that originates above the knee and crosses the joint is stretched. Flexion of the knee eliminates the action of the gastrocnemius and permits greater motion of the ankle joint (Fig. 31). Uninhibited ankle motion allows 20° dorsiflexion and 50° plantar flexion from the neutral position.

The range of motion at the ankle must be judged from the excursion of the hind foot rather than the forefoot, so that movements in the longitudinal arch are not mistaken for ankle movements (Fig. 32). Limitation of motion at the ankle joint may indicate joint or ligamentous abnormalities or gastroc-soleus contractures.

Subtalar Joint

The subtalar and transverse tarsal joints usually work together combining the movements of inversion and eversion; however, it is clinically possible to isolate the motion of each joint. The subtalar motion is tested by holding the lower leg firmly with one hand and holding the calcaneus in the other with the ankle in dorsiflexion. This ankle position fixes the talus firmly in the ankle mortise and prevents lateral motion. As the patient tries to invert then evert the foot, the motion of the heel from side to side can be palpated. This motion occurs at the subtalar joint and is

33

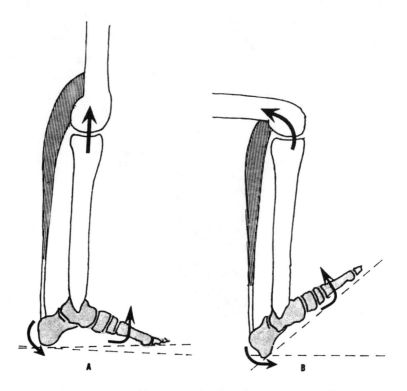

FIGURE 31. Influence of knee position on ankle plantar flexion and dorsiflexion. Because the gastrocnemius attaches above the knee joint, the ankle will not dorsiflex as much with the knee extended (A) as it does with the knee flexed (B). This mechanical factor must be kept in mind when the range of ankle motion is tested clinically.

usually 20° to either side of midline. The calcaneus can be passively moved from side to side while the other hand firmly fixes the leg.

Metatarsal Joints

Midtarsal movement is tested by grasping the heel firmly with one hand, while the other hand grasps the forefoot at the base of the metatarsals. Movement of the heel is manually prevented while the hand holding the forefoot pronates, supinates, adducts, and abducts the forefoot. The patient inverts and everts the foot voluntarily, and the range of motion is checked passively by the examiner. The range of supination motion is greater than the range of pronation. A total pronation and supination of 40° is usual.

Movements of the metatarsal bones at their proximal joints are tested individually. Because the base of the first metatarsal is kidney-shaped,

34

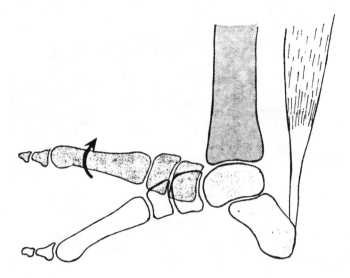

FIGURE 32. "False" impression of ankle dorsiflexion. The motion of the calcaneus indicates the range of motion. The forefoot may move upward with its movement occurring at the longitudinal arch with no elongation of the gastroc-soleus group. Clinically, the movement of the calcaneus indicates the extent of plantar flexion and dorsiflexion.

plantar flexion and dorsiflexion of this bone follow an arc about the base of the second metatarsal (Fig. 33) as it moves upon the first cuneiform.

The base of the second metatarsal bone is wedged between the medial and lateral cuneiforms (see Fig. 12) and thus moves only in one plane, that of plantar flexion and dorsiflexion. The third, fourth, and fifth metatarsals move in a plantar flexion and dorsiflexion range and arc in a rotary manner counter to the rotation of the first metatarsal. Metatarsal motion is essentially an arcuate movement in plantar flexion and dorsiflexion, the second metatarsal being fixed in one plane and the others moving in an arc around it. The end result of flexion is a transverse arcing of the metatarsals about the second metatarsal (see Fig. 33).

The range of motion of the metatarsophalangeal joint of the big toe should approach 90° of dorsiflexion; limitation to 60° or less can be considered abnormal. The big toe dorsiflexes at each step in normal walking, which subjects it to great stresses. Not only is it crowded by modern shoes, but it bears excessive body weight when high-heeled shoes are worn.

The metatarsophalangeal joint of the big toe is the site of many painful conditions such as hallux valgus, hallux rigidus, bunion, osteoarthritis, and gout, and merits careful examination in the search for the cause of pain. Full dorsiflexion (extension) of the big toe exerts traction upon the

35

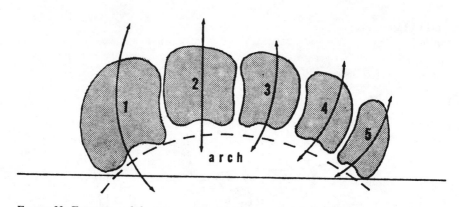

FIGURE 33. Formation of the transverse arch: movement of the individual metatarsals. The base of the second metatarsal (2) is wedged between the medial and lateral cuneiform and can only move in one plane: dorsiflexion and plantar flexion. The first metatarsal (1) moves in an arc about the second (2), and the third (3), fourth (4), and fifth (5) metatarsals arc in a contrary direction. Total plantar flexion of all the metatarsals about the pivot of the second forms the transverse arch.

plantar fascia, which simultaneously elevates the longitudinal arch of the foot (Fig. 34), a fact that should be kept in mind when plantar or calcaneal pain is being investigated.

TIBIAL ALIGNMENT

After the foot has been examined in a non-weight-bearing position and each joint individually checked, it is examined with the patient sitting

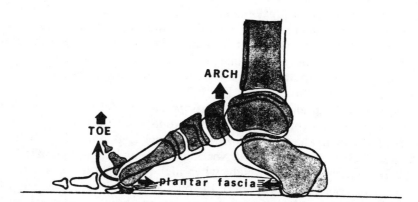

FIGURE 34. Effect of the toes upon the longitudinal arch. Full extension of the big toe exerts traction upon the plantar fascia which causes elevation of the longitudinal arch.

36

and the foot hanging freely. The patient should sit high enough so that the patient's feet are at the examiner's eye level. The leg is examined for alignment of the tibia with the knee and the ankle mortise. The tibial tuberosity should be directly under the patella and the dependent foot should invert slightly. "Tibial torsion" is a deviation in which the tibia is twisted on its longitudinal axis. With the patella in the midline, the ankle turns inward or outward depending upon the direction of the torsion. Excess torsion is most often found in infancy but its presence as a specific entity is questioned. It is frequently considered secondary to torsion of the femur. What appears to be a torsion of the tibia, may actually be a rotation at the knee in which the tibial tubercle is medial or lateral to the patellar midline (Fig. 35). These are usually familial congenital conditions that cause a "pigeon toeing" or a "Charley Chaplin" type of gait or stance.

FEMORAL ANTEVERSION

The tibia was examined for "torsion" when the patient was seated. Now the alignment of the entire lower extremity is examined while the

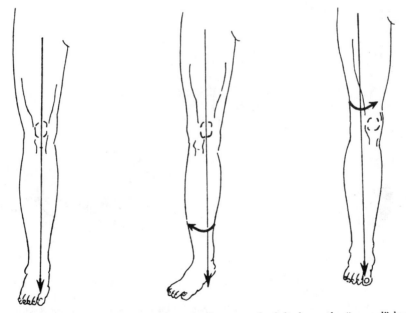

FIGURE 35. Tibial and femoral torsion. The figure to the left shows the "normal" leg in which a plumb line transects the patella and touches the foot between the first and second toes. The middle figure depicts external torsion of the leg with the tibial tubercle being externally placed to the plumb line. The figure on the right depicts internal femoral torsion.

patient is standing. A plumb line from the midpoint of the patella should drop to a point between the first and second metatarsals (see Fig. 35).

Deviations from normal alignment may indicate rotation of the femur, the tibia, or both. Excessive rotation may be congenital or an abnormality acquired during early life. The relationship of the femoral neck to the transverse axis is called the *angle of anteversion* (Fig. 36). The transcondylar axis represents a plane passing side by side through the femur. The normal range of anteversion is 15 to 25°. An increase in this angle is an increase in anteversion and results in *internal femoral torsion*. This causes "toeing-in" during walking. Techniques for measuring femoral anteversion present radiologic difficulties and have not yet been standardized.

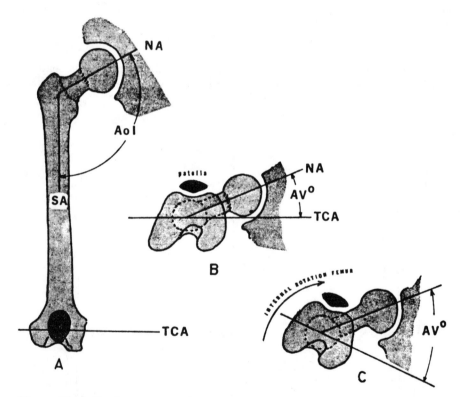

FIGURE 36. Angle of anteversion. The transcondylar axis (TCA) is a transverse line passing through the femoral condyles. An axis placed through the femoral neck (NA) forms an angle with TCA which is called the *angle of anteversion*. This is angle AV° in figure *B* with the femoral head viewed from above. A 15 to 25° angle is considered normal. In *C*, the angle is increased due to internal rotation of the femur in relationship to the femoral neck. This is increased anteversion. Viewing the femur from anterior-posterior direction, *A* depicts the *angle of inclination* (see Fig. 37). SA = angle of shaft; AoI = angle of inversion.

38

Genu varum (bowleg) and genu valgum (knock-knees) are conditions common in children. Causes must be sought when these conditions are marked or persist after infancy. Possible causes include injuries, osteomalacia, Paget's disease, or congenital variations. Congenital deviation occurs at the femoral neck in its *angle of inclination* (Fig. 37). The angle of inclination of the femoral neck is an angle formed by an axis through the femoral shaft and an axis through the neck of the femur. The normal angle varies between 116 and 140° with a greater angle forming *coxa valga* and a lesser angle *coxa vara*.

CIRCULATION

The status of the circulation is determined by noting the warmth or coolness of the skin, and the presence or absence of edema, dependent cyanosis, and blanching of the elevated foot. An ischemic foot will often

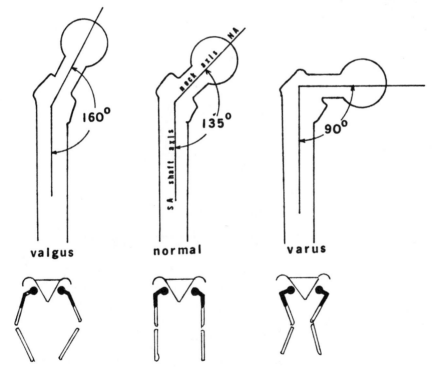

FIGURE 37. Angle of inclination. The angle formed by intersecting the femoral neck angle (NA) with an axis drawn through the shaft (SA) of the femur is termed the *angle of inclination*. This angle normally varies between 116 to 140° with the average being 135°.

39

blanch when elevated, flush when dependent, and have a thin inelastic skin lacking hair growth on the dorsum of the proximal toes. A deficient arterial blood supply is suspected when the foot becomes cyanotic on dependency and blanches on elevation.

Pitting edema noted at the end of the day and absent after a night's recumbency implies venous insufficiency. Visible varicosities enhance the diagnosis but edema, even in the presence of visible varicosities, must always raise the possibility of a systemic condition or local muscular inactivity. Poor muscular function in the lower extremity will enhance venous stasis as surely as prolonged dependence.

Palpation of arterial pulsations is the most significant test of the arterial circulation. The dorsalis pedis artery (see Fig. 27) is felt on the dorsum of the foot, between the first and second metatarsal bones (Fig. 38). The posterior tibial artery is palpable below and behind the medial malleolus of the ankle (Fig. 39). A history of claudication in which the calf cramps after walking and is relieved by rest suggests arterial insufficiency. Claudication may be induced by controlled exercise in the office and will confirm the clinical history. Claudication is also suggested when walking a specified distance causes cramping or aching in the buttocks. Known as

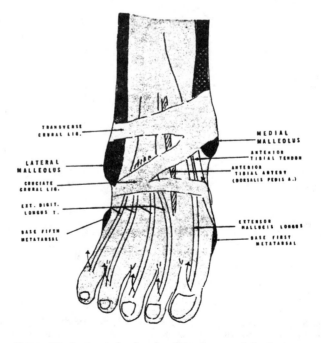

FIGURE 38. Anatomic landmarks of the dorsum of the foot.

40

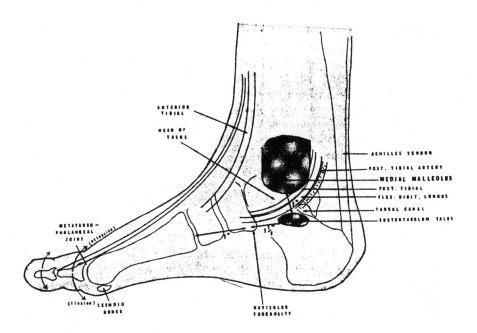

FIGURE 39. Anatomic landmarks of the medial aspect of the foot.

the LaReich syndrome, this implies occlusive vascular disease in the more proximal circulation.

Tests to determine the adequacy of circulation include measurement of skin temperature with or without contralateral limb cooling or heating, response to intra-arterial Priscoline or other vasodilators, arteriography, and oscillometry. Such tests are in the domain of the vascular specialist, but the examiner should suspect arterial insufficiency as a possible diagnosis. Oscillometry, in which pulsations are graded by an inflated cuff, may traumatize arteriosclerotic vessels causing thrombosis and emboli and does not belong in the armamentarium of the general practitioner.

NEUROLOGIC EXAMINATION

A neurologic examination should be performed on the non-weight-bearing foot by testing the Achilles reflex, knee reflex, Babinski and other upper motor neuron toe signs, and by the mapping of sensory dermatome areas. Pin scratching along the foot and leg will reveal dermatome areas of hypalgesia or anesthesia corresponding to nerve root or peripheral nerve patterns (see Fig. 27).

41

Motor Function

Motor testing is essential to the neurologic examination. The sciatic nerve, which arises from the L_4 to the S_2 spinal segments, supplies motor function of the foot and ankle. Below the knee, the sciatic nerve divides into the common peroneal nerve and the posterior tibial nerve (see Fig. 26). Since each muscle group has a specific innervation, the integrity of its nerve supply can be established by testing each muscle against manual resistance. The nerve supply can be further differentiated as a specific *root* or specific *peripheral nerve* establishing the site of nerve impairment.

The integrity of the tendons can also be determined during the test for muscle strength. Pain that may arise from the tendons will be localized during this phase of the examination. The anterior tibialis tendon crosses the medial aspect of the dorsum of the foot and can be visualized and palpated anterior to the medial malleolus when the foot is actively dorsiflexed and inverted. It is usually large and prominent. Ankle dorsiflexion and inversion are also assisted by the extensor hallucis longus (Table-1), which is primarily an extensor of the big toe. The tendon is smaller and lies on the lateral side of the anterior tibialis tendon. Its action can be eliminated by having the patient simultaneously flex the big toe while dorsiflexing the foot. The extensor hallucis longus tendon can be traced to the big toe, whereas the anterior tibial tendon disappears at the medial aspect of the foot near the base of the first metatarsal.

The extensor digitorum communis tendons can be seen and felt on the lateral aspect of the dorsum of the foot as they extend to the four outer toes. They become prominent in dorsiflexion of the toes, which is their primary function, but they also assist in dorsiflexion and eversion of the foot. In forceful ankle dorsiflexion, the anterior tibialis muscle, the extensor hallucis longus, and the extensor digitorum longus all can be seen to work simultaneously.

The plantar flexors of the foot and ankle can be tested manually, but the gastroc-soleus group is so powerful that the only true test of strength and endurance is to have the patient repeatedly rise on the tiptoes of each foot individually to watch for weakness and fatigue. The extensibility of the calf muscles should be determined by passive dorsiflexion of the foot

TABLE 1. Nerve and Muscle Relationship in Dorsiflexion of the Foot and Ankle

Muscle Supplied	Origin	Nerve
Tibialis anterior	L_4, L_5, S_1	deep peroneal nerve branch of
Extensor digitorum longus	L_5, S_1	the common peroneal nerve
Extensor hallucis longus	L_5, S_1	

TABLE 2. Nerve and Muscle Relationship in Plantar Flexion of the Foot and Ankle

Muscle Supplied	Origin	Nerve
Gastrocnemius	S_1, S_2	
Soleus	L_5, S_1, S_2	
Tibialis posterior	L_5, S_1	Tibial
Flexor digitorum longus	L_5, S_1	
Flexor hallucis longus	L_5, S_1	
Peroneus longus and brevis	L_5, S_1	Superficial peroneal nerve (branch of the common peroneal nerve)

with the knee extended, watching the excursion of the calcaneus, and noting any limitation of motion (see Fig. 32). The degree of ankle dorsiflexion with the knee flexed establishes the elongation of the soleus muscle (see Fig. 31). The markedly everted pronated foot usually has a shortened Achilles tendon and limitation of dorsiflexion; therefore, to accurately measure dorsiflexion, the foot should be held in slight inversion by the examiner.

Plantar flexion of the foot and ankle is assisted by the tibialis posterior, the toe flexors, and the peroneus longus and brevis (Table-2). The principal function of these muscles can be tested individually.

Inversion of the foot is initiated by the tibialis anterior muscle, and the extensor hallucis longus as their tendons insert on the inner border of the forefoot. The gastrocnemius and soleus *invert* the foot. When the foot is flat on the floor and weight-bearing, the Achilles tendon elevates the calcaneus. This motion occurs about the subtalar axis and causes supination of the forefoot.

The tibialis posterior is the major invertor of the foot and is innervated by the posterior tibialis nerve (see Fig. 26). Its tendon can be palpated behind and below the medial malleolus when the foot is actively inverted and plantar flexed (see Fig. 39).

Eversion of the foot is initiated by the extensor digitorum longus when the foot is in the neutral or dorsiflexion position, but in plantar flexion the peroneus longus and brevis initiate the major eversion action. The peronei receive their nerve supply from the superficial peroneal nerve (see Fig. 26), and their tendons can be palpated behind and below the lateral malleolus (Fig. 40).

The four layers of the intrinsic muscles of the sole of the foot were discussed briefly in Chapter 1 (see Figs. 20 to 23). They are innervated by the medial and lateral plantar nerves (see Fig. 24) and function primarily to arch the sole of the foot in a "cupping" motion.

The gross appearance of the non-weight-bearing foot is observed noting its color and skin texture. Calluses are noted and related to the underlying

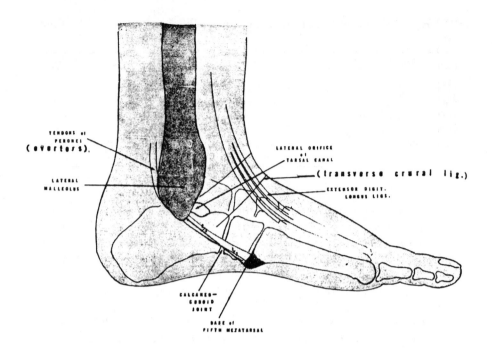

FIGURE 40. Superficial anatomic landmarks of the lateral aspect of the foot.

bone structure. Corns and calluses are found at the sites of pain and examination reveals the underlying cause. They occur at sites of faulty weight bearing or pressures during stance or walking, and usually indicate improper shoe fit.

The weight-bearing foot is now examined. A footprint gives an indication of weight-bearing points and surfaces. The longitudinal arch is checked with the patient standing. If the inner border of the foot is in contact with the floor a "flatfoot" is indicated.

FLATFOOT

The *flatfoot* is common and has many varied types. The flatfoot due to a fat pad under the arch, is noted so frequently in infants as to be considered normal and will be discussed in Chapter 5. If the lower limb is angulated either at the femur or the tibia, the foot will pronate because the line of weight bearing falls inside the normal midline (see Fig. 35) and places undue stress upon the longitudinal arch. "Knock-knees" in children cause a shift in the center of gravity that may cause the foot to bear weight on its inner margin and thus flatten the foot.

44

Relaxed Flatfoot

A relaxed flatfoot has a good longitudinal arch that disappears upon weight bearing and usually reforms when the patient rises on the toes. This condition implies ligamentous laxity and may be congenital. It often arises in middle-aged individuals in occupations that require prolonged standing. It also occurs in people who have gained excessive weight, received inadequate exercise, or experienced a period of prlonged bed rest. It need not be symptomatic and treatment is not always indicated.

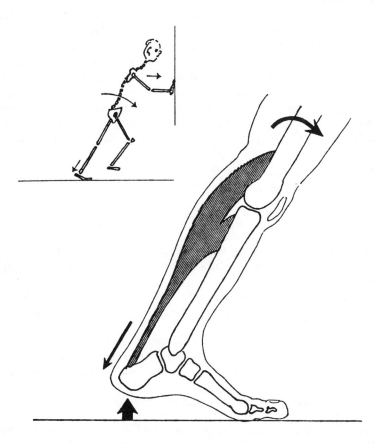

FIGURE 41. Testing Achilles tendon elongation in the erect position. The patient stands away from the wall and leans against it. The leg to be tested remains behind with the knee extended and the heel against the floor. The other leg is brought forward, the knee bent, and the foot elevated. The Achilles tendon is stretched as the body leans forward. The heel will rise from the floor if the Achilles is shortened, and characteristic pain can be reproduced. This movement may also be used as an exercise to stretch the heel cord.

In very severe flatfoot, the navicular and the head of the talus are in contact with the ground and the head of the talus is very prominent. The heel and forefoot are usually everted, and the forefoot is splayed.

Rigid Flatfoot

The rigid flatfoot is a pronated foot with an inflexible depressed arch and implies soft tissue contracture, articular damage, unreduced fracture or dislocation, or bony ankylosis. A rigid flatfoot can result from fibrous contracture of the peronei muscles. X-ray examination may be necessary to differentiate the cause of the rigid flatfoot.

The Achilles tendon was tested for shortening during an earlier phase of the examination with the knee extended to test the gastrocnemius, and the knee flexed to test the soleus (see Figs. 31 and 32). Achilles tendon shortening also can be tested by having the patient keep the knees straight and the heels in contact with the floor, while leaning forward against a wall. This stretches the Achilles tendon. The leg being tested remains in this position as the other leg is brought forward, with the knee bent and the foot elevated. The heel will rise from the floor if the Achilles tendon is shortened. Complaints of calf pain can be reproduced by this procedure (Fig. 41).

The examination is completed by observing foot performance during walking both with and without shoes.

BIBLIOGRAPHY

ADAMS, JC: *Outline of Orthopaedics,* ed 5. Williams & Wilkins, Baltimore, 1964.

BAILEY, H: *Demonstrations of Physical Signs in Clinical Surgery,* ed 13. Williams & Wilkins, Baltimore, 1960.

GARTLAND, JJ: Fundamentals of Orthopaedics. WB Saunders, Philadelphia, 1965.

HAYMAKER, W AND WOODHALL, B: *Peripheral Nerve Injuries: Principles of Diagnosis,* ed 2. WB Saunders, Philadelphia, 1959.

LEWIN, P: *The Foot and Ankle,* ed 4. Lea & Febiger, Philadelphia, 1959.

MILGRAM, JE: *Office measures for relief of the painful foot.* J Bone Joint Surg 46:1095, 1964.

OESTER, YT AND MAYER, JH, JR: *Motor Examination of Peripheral Nerve Injuries.* Charles C Thomas, Springfield, Ill, 1960.

RYDER, CT AND CRANE, L: *Measuring femoral anteversion: The problem and a method.* J Bone Joint Surg 35-A:321, 1953.

SCHWARTZ, RP AND HEATH, AL: *Pointed and round-toed shoes.* J Bone Joint Surg 48-A:2, 1966.

WILSON, JN: *The treatment of deformities of the foot and toes.* British Journal of Physical Medicine 17:73 (April) 1954.

CHAPTER 3

The Foot During Walking

To understand the role of the foot and ankle, all the components of man's gait must be evaluated. Observations on the mechanics of walking were recorded as far back as Aristotle and Leonardo da Vinci, and in recent decades all components of walking have been studied with great scientific precision. The search for better prosthetic devices for war amputees has placed an emphasis on the study of gait *biomechanics* in this century. Three-dimensional views of gait have been analyzed by the combined use of cameras, mirrors, and electromyography. The energy expended by individual muscles in all phases of gait is being investigated to determine their contribution.

Static deformities and pathologic gaits can be better understood through a thorough knowledge of normal gait. The role of the foot and ankle must be studied within all the determinants of gait.

Locomotion is the translation of the body from one point to another. Initiation of locomotion requires an interplay between the forces of gravity, inertia, and the ground as affected by the contraction of muscles acting upon the lower extremities. Human locomotion has been compared to a wheel rolling over the ground with the legs being two of its spokes. The spoke that touches the ground constitutes the "stance" phase of walking, and the spoke that moves about the axle is the "swing" phase.

If the axis of the wheel moves in a horizontal line, a minimum of energy is expended in accordance with *Newton's law of motion* which states that "a body will continue to move in a straight line unless a contrary force impells a change." All the determinants of gait minimize the forces that tend to impede effortless motion. In essence, man attempts to keep his center of gravity moving in a straight horizontal line during locomotion.

Man's center of gravity is located just anterior to his second sacral vertebra, midway between both hip joints. Walking is initiated by inclining the body forward thus placing it ahead of its center of gravity. To regain balance, one leg must be brought forward ahead of the shifting center of gravity. The leg that remains weight bearing is the "stance" leg and must always be in contact with the ground. The leg that moves to regain balance is the "swing" limb.

The stance leg as it remains to the rear of the center of gravity helps to propel the body forward. Walking therefore can be divided into a "stance" phase, in which a leg is weight-bearing, and a "swing" phase, in which the leg is moved to another point of contact. The stance phase occupies about 60 percent of the *gait cycle,* which begins as the heel strikes the ground and ends after the swing phase has again found the same heel "striking."

During the early 10 percent and late 10 percent of the stance phase, both feet are on the ground and both legs are in a stance phase. After 10 percent of stance phase, the opposite leg is in its swing phase and there ensues a single-leg support phase.

In Figure 42, at 0 percent, the heel of the stance foot is on the ground, but by 7 percent the foot is flat upon the ground. The activity occurs rapidly in the gait cycle. This stance phase of double-leg support lasts about 12 percent of the gait cycle, by which time the other leg enters the swing phase until 50 percent of the gait. This phase, 12 to 50 percent, is obviously a single-leg phase; one weight-bearing and the other swing.

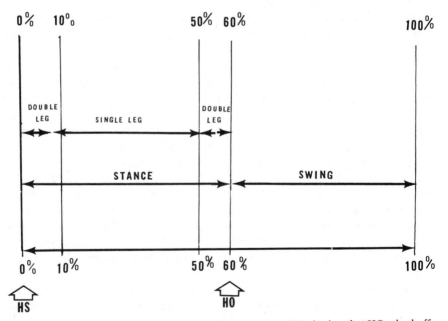

FIGURE 42. Analysis of gait: Single- and double-leg phases. HS - heel strike; HO - heel-off.

At 60 to 62 percent of the walking cycle, the stance leg begins heel-off (originally termed toe-off) and that leg begins swing phase while the other leg is in a single-leg stance phase.

The body, and thus the leg and foot have impact upon the ground that has been measured by force plates (Fig. 43). There are three forces: (1) vertical, (2) shear in a horizontal, forward, and backward direction as related to the ground, and (3) torque, transverse rotation of the limb to the ground.

At initial contact (heel strike) the force of 70 percent of the body weight is imparted to the foot. As the leg is flexed at the point of the gait cycle (see Fig. 43) the center of gravity is at its lowest point. As the gait progresses, the foot flattens to the ground and the leg extends at the hip, elevating the center of gravity. The weight supported on raising the body is in the vicinity of 110 to 125 percent of body weight.

At 30 percent of the gait cycle, when the body is single-leg supported, with that leg flat-footed and the leg extended but the knee slightly flexed, the vertical force is about 75 percent of body weight. This drop in vertical force is probably due to the change in the vertical elevation of the center

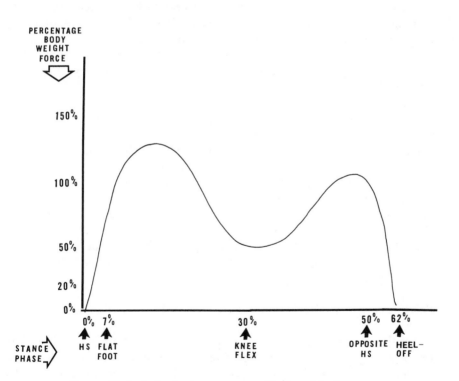

FIGURE 43. Analysis of gait: percentage of body weight force.

49

of gravity with a beginning descent (drop) of the center of gravity. By 50 percent of the gait cycle, the opposite leg enters full strike and the center of gravity is again low; the percentage of body weight vertical force drops to less than half of the body weight.

GAIT DETERMINANTS

If man were to walk with his knees stiff and his pelvis moving in a straight line, his center of gravity would describe a high, undulating pathway. Its highest point would occur when the stiff weight-bearing leg was vertical (mid-stance) and its lowest when one limb is fully flexed and the other extended at the hip (double-leg stance) (Fig. 44). This type of gait would be jerky and require a great deal of energy to alternately elevate and depress the body weight at each step. Man does not walk this way but normally uses various movements of his hips, knees, ankles, and pelvis to maintain his center of gravity on a horizontally level plane. These movements are known as *determinants of gait;* together they increase efficiency, decrease energy expenditure, and make the gait more graceful.

During a complete cycle, the center of gravity is displaced twice in its vertical axis. The peak occurs during the middle of the stance phase when the weight-bearing leg is vertical and its lowest point when both legs are weight-bearing with one at the position of *heel strike* and the other at *heel-off.* The undulating center of gravity may transcribe a cycle that has a vertical displacement of 2 inches.

Pelvic Rotation

Decrease of the height of the vertical undulations is attempted by *pelvic rotation* in which the pelvis oscillates about an axis of the lumbar spine. Viewed from above, one side of the pelvis comes forward with the limb that is swinging forward. This movement lessens the angle between the pelvis and the thigh, which also lessens the angle between the leg and the floor. The extent that the pelvis depresses during the step is also decreased (Fig. 45). The pelvis rotates approximately 4° on each side, with a total rotation of 8°, and by this rotation, the vertical undulation of the center of gravity is decreased by 3/8 inch.

Pelvic Tilt

Another determinant of gait is *pelvic tilt* (Fig. 46), a drop of the pelvis on the swing side. The stance leg at this point is adducted, and the swinging leg is slightly abducted (Fig. 47) and flexed at the hip and knee to clear the floor. This flexion with the simultaneous "Trendelenburg posi-

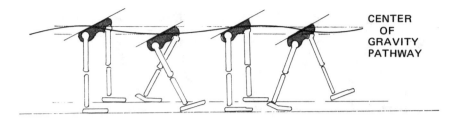

FIGURE 44. Undulant course of pelvic center in gait without determinants. The marked vertical undulations of the center of gravity occur when gait is performed with stiff knees and no lateral motion of the pelvis.

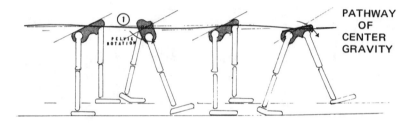

FIGURE 45. Pelvic rotation: first determinant of gait. The pelvis rotates forward with the "swinging" leg thus decreasing the angle formed by the leg with the floor and at the hip joint. This rotation decreases the vertical undulations of the center of gravity of the pelvis.

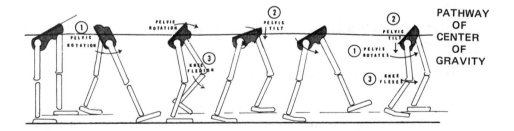

FIGURE 46. Pelvic tilt: second determinant of gait. Pelvic rotation is shown in 1. As the left leg swings through, the pelvis on the left drops (2), and the left hip and knee flex (3). The figure on the right shows the right let swinging through with the right side of the pelvis dipping and the right hip and knee flexing.

51

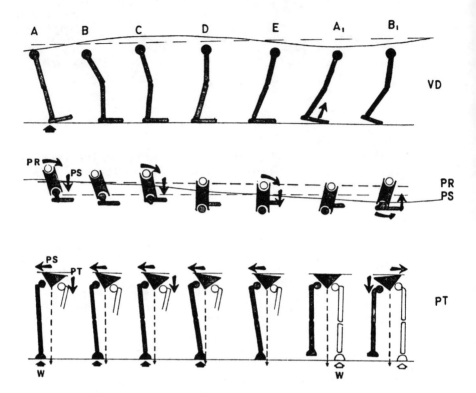

FIGURE 47. Composite of first two determinants of gait. VD shows vertical displacement from the side view. PR is pelvic rotation as the leg swings through. PT indicates pelvic tilt. The bottom figures illustrate gait from the front and show lateral shift of the pelvis combined with tilt and rotation. The weight-bearing leg (W), goes into a "Trendelenburg position": adducting as the pelvis shifts over it. The swinging leg is slightly abducted. PS indicates pelvic shift and the arrows the direction of the shift.

tion" of the other hip decreases the vertical undulation by an additional 1/8 inch.

Knee Flexion During Stance Phase

The third determinant of gait is *knee flexion* during the stance phase. The knee is fully extended at heel strike which starts the stance phase for that leg. As the body moves over its center of gravity, the knee flexes (Fig. 48) approximately 15° until the foot is flat upon the ground. The body then passes over the foot, and the knee gradually re-extends to full extension at the end of the stance phase. This knee flexion decreases the extent of pelvic undulation by an additional 1/8 inch.

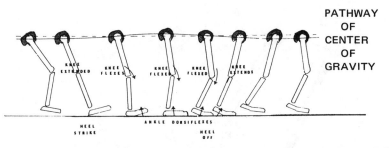

FIGURE 48. Knee flexion during stance phase: third determinant of gait. The knee is fully extended at heel strike. As the body passes over the center of gravity, the knee flexes to decrease the vertical amplitude of the pathway of the center of gravity. The knee re-extends at the end of the stance phase: the "heel-off."

Knee-Ankle Relationship

The fourth determinant upon gait is a combined *motion of the knee and ankle*. This knee action, although similar to the third determinant, is different in relating principally to ankle motion in its influence upon the pathway of pelvic undulation. At heel strike, the ankle is dorsiflexed to about 90° and gradually plantar flexes to become flat on the ground as the body approaches the center of gravity. This rotation occurs about the ankle joint. As the ankle joint passes over the weight-bearing heel, two small arcs of motion occur which the knee, by slight flexion, smooths out (Fig. 49).

Pelvic Shift

A last determinant is *pelvic shift* in which the pelvis moves laterally to maintain body balance as one leg is lifted from the ground. As the pelvis shifts, the weight-bearing limb adducts (see Fig. 47). This sway from side to side smooths the pelvic movement as well as maintaining balance.

Interactions of Determinants

The determinants of pelvic rotation, pelvic tilting, knee and ankle flexion, and pelvic shift all aim to decrease the amplitude of vertical displacement of the pelvis and to decrease the degree of undulation. Both of these decrease the energy required to raise and lower the body during walking.

A flattened pathway in the vertical displacement increases the *relative* length of the lower extremity, thus increasing the length of the stride without increasing the degree of hip flexion and extension. As the speed of locomotion is dependent upon the length of the stride rather than an

53

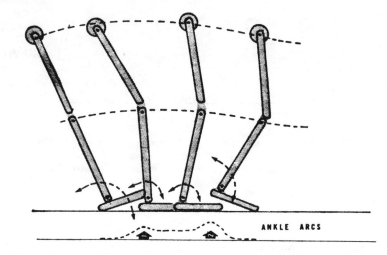

ANKLE ARCS

FIGURE 49. Foot and ankle relationship: fourth determinant of gait. At the heel strike the ankle is dorsiflexed 90°. The level of the ankle rises slightly as the foot goes forward into the "flatfoot stance" phase. This is followed by the ankle again dorsiflexing as the leg passes over the foot. At push-off the heel rises giving a second small upward undulation. These two small undulations at the ankle are *smoothed out* by simultaneous knee flexions.

increase in cadence, the determinants of gait improve forward velocity, without increasing gait cadence and thus further conserve energy.

TRANSVERSE ROTATION

The above determinants concern motion of the lower extremity in a sagittal plane. During locomotion, there is a transverse rotation of the lower extremity which also facilitates gait. In addition to the rotation of the pelvis, which has been mentioned, the thigh, leg, and ankle also rotate about the longitudinal axis.

As the limb begins its swing phase, the femur begins to rotate internally, and simultaneously the tibia rotates internally upon the femur. This rotation continues past heel strike into the stance phase and ends when the foot is fully flat upon the ground. It is at this point that the opposite leg begin its swing phase and its internal rotation.

Once the foot is flat, derotation begins as the pelvis passes over the fixed weight-bearing foot. Simultaneously, the stance hip and tibia gradually rotate externally. Any rotation in the foot must occur at the subtalar joint because the foot is fixed to the floor and no latter motion is permitted at the ankle mortise.

54

PLANTAR FASCIA

The plantar fascia (see Fig. 25) passively functions during gait in a mechanical manner. It arises from the anterior portion of the calcaneus and, as it passes forward, attaches to the base of the proximal phalanges and simultaneously attaches to the overlying skin (Fig. 50). The plantar fascia varies in thickness, being thickest in its mid-portion and thinning medially and laterally.

The fibers of the plantar fascia at the ball of the foot are arranged in transverse bands, longitudinal bands, and vertical fibers. This intertwining of fibers, forms compartments that contain fat to protect the nerves and blood vessels as they pass through the compartments (Fig. 51). The vertical fibers connect the skin to the skeletal boney structures.

When the foot is in a relaxed state, the pad under the metatarsal heads is soft and pliable, and the overlying skin moveable. During walking or running, the ball of the foot is exposed not only to heavy pressures, but also to forceful traction forces. This places stress upon the skin and the subcutaneous tissues, and compresses the tissues about the nerves and blood vessels as they pass from the sole to the digits. As the toe extends (dorsiflexes upward), the pad *and* the skin become taut and tense. This occurs because of the distal attachments of the plantar fascia (Fig. 52). There are bursae between the metatarsal heads (see Fig. 51) that protect the heads and the underlying compartmental contents (nerves, blood vessels, and lumbricals). In conditions such as Morton's neuralgia (see Chapter 11), the bursal inflammation and swelling may well contribute to the symptoms attributable to the neuritis.

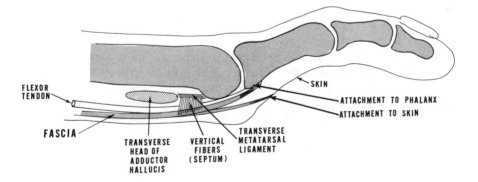

FIGURE 50. Lateral view of the plantar fascial attachments. Attachment of the distal fibers of the fascia to the proximal phalanx (along with the flexor tendon) and to the skin. The vertical fibers form the septum depicted in Figure 51.

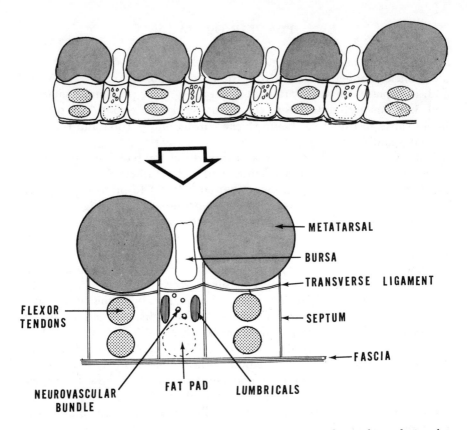

FIGURE 51. Schematic view of fascial metatarsal compartments. The top figure depicts the compartments formed by the plantar fascial fibers, with the longitudinal fibers forming tunnels. The flexor tendons pass through the tunnels, under the metatarsal bones and parallel compartments, which contain nerves, blood vessels, and lumbricals. The intermetatarsal bursae are shown.

The plantar fascia has been termed a "windlass mechanism" (Hicks) (Fig. 53). As the toes dorsiflex during gait in heel-off to toe-off, the plantar pads wind around the metatarsal heads and raise the longitudinal arch. The medial aspect of the plantar fascia is mechanically more efficient than is the lateral, and may contribute to supinating the foot.

TALONAVICULAR JOINT

The talonavicular joint also has mechanical factors that stabilize the joint. The convexity of the head of the talus differs in regard to the plane in which it is observed. Viewed from the superior aspect, the curvature is broader than when viewed laterally. This asymmetry stabilizes the medial

56

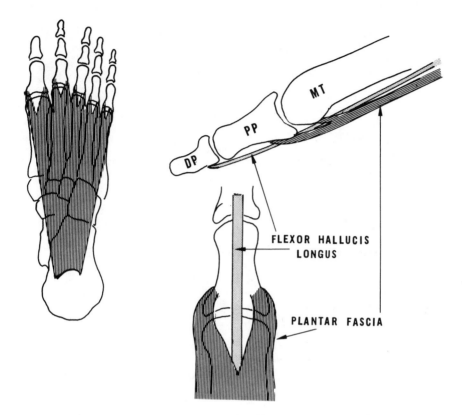

FIGURE 52. Distal attachment of the plantar fascia and flexor hallucis longus tendon.

aspect of the foot, particularly at the end of the stance phase when the heel-off proceeds to toe-off and the foot undergoes supination.

FOOT ANGULATION

The average angle of "toe-out" of the weight-bearing foot to the plane of forward progression is usually 6 to 7° (Fig. 54). A greater degree of toeing out occurs in the aged and improves balance. In faster walking, stability is less of a problem and toeing out decreases to the point of being totally eliminated.

MUSCULAR ACTION

Locomotion depends upon muscles as movers, stabilizers, and decelerators. Muscles of the lower extremity may act across one or two joints.

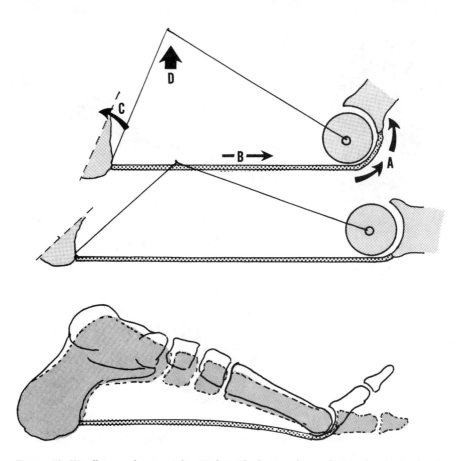

FIGURE 53. Windlass mechanism (after Hicks). The bottom figure depicts the plantar fascia with toe plantar flexed (shaded area) and the higher arch with the toe dorsiflexed (clear area). The top figure shows how the plantar fascia winds around the metatarsal head and during dorsiflexion *(A)* places tension upon the fascia *(B)*, altering the angle of the calcaneus *(C)* and elevation of the longitudinal arch *(D)*.

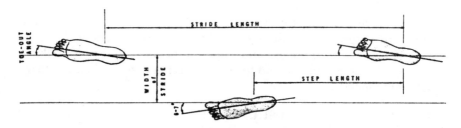

FIGURE 54. Outward angulation of the feet during walking. A "toe-out" angle of 6 to 7° is usual but increases with aging. Faster walking decreases the toe-out angle to 0°. Length of stride is measured from stance of the foot to the next stance of the same foot.

58

They may move a free segment of the extremity or act from a fixed segment.

Walking can begin with relaxation of the *gastroc-soleus* group to permit a forward inclination of the body ahead of the center of gravity (see Fig. 18). With this shift forward, the supporting foot becomes the *propulsive* foot. The weight-bearing portion of the foot shifts from the heel, along the lateral side of the foot, and across the metatarsal heads toward the pad of the big toe (Fig. 55). The big toe presses the ground stabilizing the foot and aiding in the push-off.

Major muscular activity begins during the last 10° of the swing phase and ends after the first 10° of the stance phase. From the activity occurring at the *end of the swing phase*, it is apparent that muscular activity decelerates the limb rather than combating gravity. After heel strike, the body is "pulled forward" over the anchored foot. During the stance phase, the *calf muscles* act almost exclusively to decelerate the leg as it

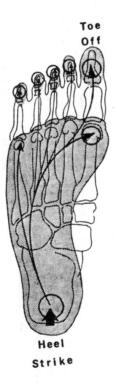

Toe Off

Heel Strike

FIGURE 55. Path of weight bearing of the foot during walking. Weight bearing begins at the heel *(heel strike)* and proceeds along the lateral border of the foot toward the metatarsal heads with the major propulsive thrust by the distal phalanx of the big toe *(heel-off)*.

59

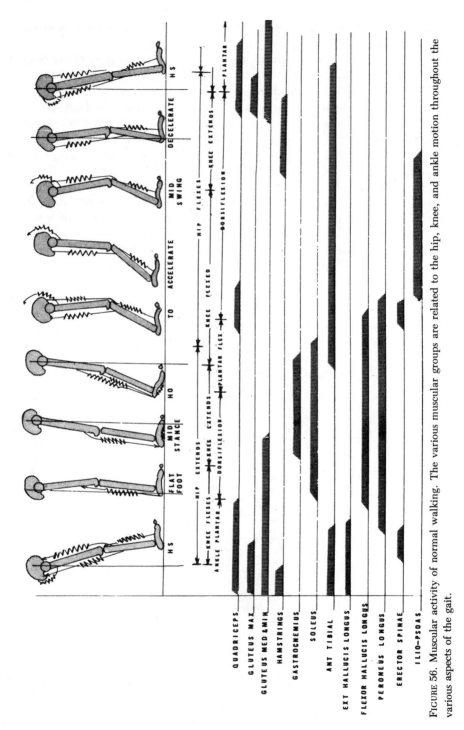

FIGURE 56. Muscular activity of normal walking. The various muscular groups are related to the hip, knee, and ankle motion throughout the various aspects of the gait.

60

passes over the foot (Fig. 56). Sixty percent of energy expended is used for deceleration rather than propulsion against gravity.

Muscular activity during gait is depicted in Figures 56 and 57. The *erector spinae* muscles raise the pelvis, and the *glutei* stabilize the hip during lateral pelvic shifting. The *hip flexors* initiate the swing phase, but the impetus of the swinging limb is delivered by the pendular extension of the leg upon the thigh. The *quadriceps*, which acts across two joints, flexes the hip while simultaneously extending the knee when the foot is free. It is during the "swing through" that the thigh and leg rotate inwardly.

Early in the swing phase, the *hamstring* muscles flex the knee if a faster cadence is needed. At the end of the swing phase (see Fig. 57), the hamstring muscles brake the swinging lower limb to minimize the impact of knee extension. The *pretibial* group of muscles is active throughout the entire swing phase to raise the toes to clear the floor. Immediately after heel strike, the ankle dorsiflexors brake the plantar motion of the foot to prevent a forceful foot "slap" (Figs. 57 and 58).

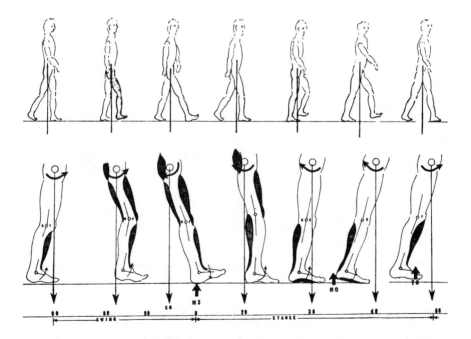

FIGURE 57. Muscular activity of the lower extremity during normal gait. The muscular activity as viewed in the right leg is shown through a complete stride cycle.

61

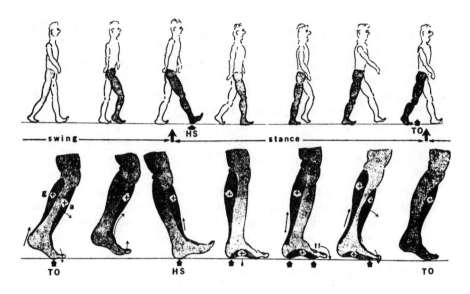

FIGURE 58. Muscular activity of the leg and ankle during normal gait. This duplicates Figure 57 but concentrates upon the leg, ankle, and foot during gait from toe-off through a full stride.

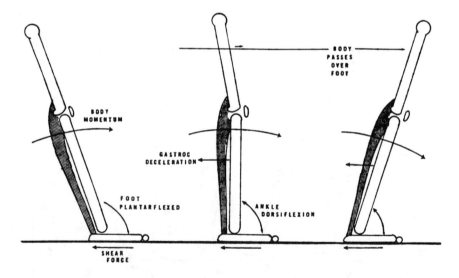

FIGURE 59. Ankle dorsiflexion during stance phase of gait. The ankle dorsiflexes during stance phase by mechanical forces. As the leg passes over the foot the ankle is dorsiflexed *without* action of the dorsiflexor muscles. The gastroc-soleus group is active throughout this action and acts to *decelerate* the forward motion of the body. The floor applies a *shear stress* to the foot during this action.

The *plantar flexors* remain active during the middle and last portions of the stance phase. As the heel leaves the ground the plantar flexors cease all activity. Throughout most of the stance phase, as the leg passes over the foot, the ankle is dorsiflexing upon the tibia. During this dorsiflexion, the pretibial muscles are inactive and the plantar flexors are contracting. This indicates that dorsiflexion of the ankle is achieved mechanically and the gastroc-soleus group is used for deceleration (Figs. 57 to 59).

Shortly after heel strike, when the foot has become flat against the ground, the lower limb begins to rotate externally. The foot is now fixed on the ground so rotation of the leg and foot occurs at the subtalar joint and causes the foot to supinate (Figs. 60 and 61). This subtalar rotation aligns the Achilles tendon more centrally, and thus gives the plantar flexors more efficiency and the foot more stability.

The foot during walking can be better understood when studied in relationship to the total biomechanics of the lower limb during gait.

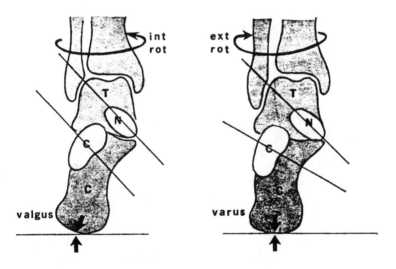

FIGURE 60. Supination of the foot during external rotation of the leg. With the foot weight-bearing during stance phase, external rotation of the leg causes the foot to rotate at the subtalar joint and *supinate* the foot. The leg begins to externally rotate during walking when the foot is fully flat against the floor. The supinated position places the calcaneus into more varus and thus places the Achilles tendon in a more direct alignment with the leg. With the everted calcaneus (valgus), the transverse tarsal axies are parallel allowing flexibility; whereas in the varus heel position, the axies are not parallel and the foot becomes rigid. In the foot during walking, the heel is in varus at heel strike and in valgus at mid-stance to resume varus at toe-off.

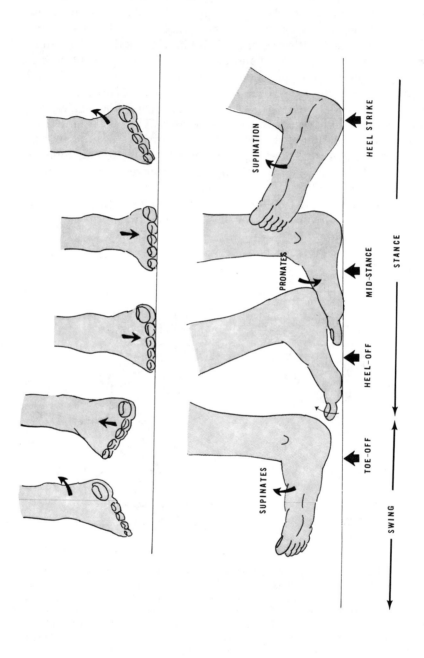

FIGURE 61. Foot during stance phase. From heel strike to flatfoot this occurs at 7 percent of stance phase through 12 percent; at 35 percent the heel leaves the floor (heel-off). Toe-off starts the swing phase of that leg and begins at 60 percent of stance phase.

BIBLIOGRAPHY

BASMAJIAN, JV: *Man's Posture*. Archives of Physical Medicine 46:26, 1965.

BASMAJIAN, JV AND STECKO, G: *The roles of muscles in arch support of the foot*. J Bone Joint Surg 45-A:1184, 1963.

BOJSEN-MOLLER, F AND FLAGSTAD, KE: *Plantar aponeurosis and internal architecture of the ball of the foot*. J Anat 121(3):599, 1976.

BRANTINGHAM, CR, EGGE, AS, AND BEEKMAN, BE: *The effect of artificially varied surface on ambulatory rehabilitation with preliminary EMG evaluation of certain muscles involved*. Presented at APA Annual Meeting, Los Angeles, August 1963.

HICKS, JH: *The three weight-bearing mechanisms of the foot*. In EVANS, F GAYNOR (ED): *Biomechanical Studies of the Musculo-Skeletal System*. Charles C Thomas, Springfield, Ill, 1961, p 172.

LEVENS, AS, INMAN, VT, AND BLOSSER, JA: *Transverse rotation of the segments of the lower extremity in locomotion*. J Bone Joint Surg 30-A:849, 1948.

LIBERSON, WT: *Biomechanics of gait: A method of study*. Archives of Physical Medicine 46:37, 1965.

MACCONAILL, MA: *The postural mechanism of the human foot*. Proceedings of the Royal Irish Academy 1B:265, 1945.

MANN, R AND INMANN, VT: *Phasic activity of intrinsic muscles of the foot*. J Bone Joint Surg 46-A:469, 1964.

MORTON, DJ: *Human Locomotion and Body Form: A Study of Gravity and Man*. Williams & Wilkins, Baltimore, 1952.

MURRAY, MP, DROUGHT, AB, AND KORY, RC: *Walking patterns of normal men*. J Bone Joint Surg 46-A:335, 1964.

MURRAY, MP, et al: *Comparison of free and fast speed walking patterns of normal men*. Am J Phys Med 45:8, 1966.

SAUNDER, JB de CM, INMANN, VT, AND EBERHART, HD: *The major determinants in normal and pathological gait*. J Bone Joint Surg 35-A:543, 1953.

STEINDLER, A: *Kinesiology: Of the Human Body, Under Normal and Pathological Conditions*. Charles C Thomas, Springfield, 1977.

SUTHERLAND, DH: *An electromyographic study of the plantar flexors of the ankle in normal walking on the level*. J Bone Joint Surg 48-A:66, 1966.

WRIGHT, DG, DESAI, SM, AND HENDERSON, WH: *Action of the subtalar and ankle joint complex during the stance phase of walking*. Biomechanics Laboratory, University of California, San Francisco, No 38, June 1962.

65

CHAPTER 4

The Foot in Jogging and Running

The foot, as shown in Figure 57 (see Chapter 3), indicates that in walking, one third of the gait is swing and two thirds is stance, whereas in running two thirds is swing and only one third is stance.

Velocity, cadence, and stride length increase with the speed of the gait. "Floating" time (time in which neither foot contacts the ground) does not exist in walking, whereas floating time is 20 percent of the gait cycle in jogging, and 40 percent in running. The hip, knee, and ankle ranges of motion are increased as the gait increases. Due to the increase of knee flexion and increased dorsiflexion to the ankle, the center of gravity is lowered.

There is full extension of the hip in walking, but this occurs after lift-off in jogging and running caused by not enough time during the stance phase. Knee flexion at initial floor contact (heel strike) is 7° in walking and 40° in jogging and running. In walking, the knee flexes 7° at heel strike to 10° at mid-stance, whereas in jogging and running, the initial flexion goes to 60° of flexion. During walking, there is plantar flexion at initial floor contact; in jogging or running the ankle is dorsiflexed. Dorsiflexion occurs throughout the stance phase in all forms of ambulation.

FORCE

Initial impact on the ground (heel strike) is 85 percent of body weight walking, and 170 percent body weight jogging. There follows a second spike of vertical force to 100 percent in walking, 250 percent in jogging and slightly less in running. In walking, the double elevation is not apparent in the jogging and running individual as, there is no valley and no second increase of peak of center of gravity elevation. In running, it is even smoother indicating the efficience of walking due to the "float."

66

Shear Forces

The shear forces are *equal* in walking or jogging as the energy is used to elevate and descend the body in an up and down vertical manner. However, the shear forces are *double* in running. This is possibly due to the angle of the body and more energy propelling the body forward.

MUSCULAR ACTIVITY

In walking, acceleration is 20 to 30 percent of the gait. In hip extension by gluteus maximus, the hamstrings are active at the end of the swing phase, and during the first 10 percent of the stance phase after heel strike. In jogging and running, the hamstrings become active in the last 25 percent of swing phase. They remain active through two thirds of the stance phase in jogging and one half of the stance phase in running.

Quadriceps

In walking or jogging, the quadriceps is active during the late stage of swing phase and the first 15 percent of stance phase at heel strike, and early stance phase as the knee flexes. In running, the quadriceps becomes active during the last half of swing phase and the first half of stance phase.

Gastrocnemius

In walking, at mid-stance, the gastrocnemius restrains the forward movement of the tibia over the fixed foot. There is no *push-off*, only *lift-off* of the foot.

In jogging and running, however, the gastrocnemius becomes active at the end of swing phase (heel strike), and remains active through 80 percent of the stance phase in jogging and 50 percent in running. The gastrocnemius becomes immediately active upon foot-ground contact, which begins essentially at heel strike, to decelerate (i.e., to absorb shock). The gastrocnemius actually contracts, but only to 50 percent of ankle plantar flexion.

Anterior Tibialis

This muscle is active throughout the entire swing phase of walking, beginning its contraction late in the stance phase. (This is activity to clear the floor.) It also simultaneously supinates (inverts) the foot, as well as dorsiflexes the forefoot.

In walking, the anterior tibialis is active while the foot is plantar flexing, decelerating the foot drop.

In running, the anterior tibialis is active just after toe-off, and continues throughout the swing phase and the first 60 percent of the stance phase. Because of the force becoming smoothed out, it is much more efficient due primarily to the float time which is apparent in running, but not walking.

THE FOOT IN ATHLETES

As the gait in running consists of alternating single-leg support with no double-leg stance phase, running is essentially coordinated, alternating jumps from one leg to the other. There is heel strike with foot supinated, mid-support with foot slightly pronated, heel rise with foot supinated, thus, toe-off to immediate forward swing of that leg to immediate heel strike again.

INJURIES

Hamstring Strain

The hamstrings, as previously explained, become active in the last 25 percent of the swing phase in running, and remain active through two thirds of the stance phase in jogging and one half of the stance phase in running. Even though the stance phase is decreased in these activities, it indicates why hamstring strain is so common.

Painful Heel Pad

The initial impact of body weight on the heel, 170 percent in jogging and 250 percent in running, certainly indicates why a painful heel pad is so apparent in runners. Especially those who run on hard surfaces with inadequate heel padding in their shoes. At heel strike, the calcaneous contacts the ground surface with the heel fat pads cushioning the impact (Fig. 62).

In young feet, the heel pads are fat lobules encased in septal compartments. As aging occurs, the septa become thinner and the fat more liquid, thus decreasing the efficacy of the cushion. There occurs more periosteal contact with bleeding and fibrous scar formation, with resultant pain and tenderness. Treatment for this condition is to pad the heel with shock absorbent material (see Fig. 62). Hollowing out the center area that receives the impact, distributes the pressure on other portions of the calcaneus.

68

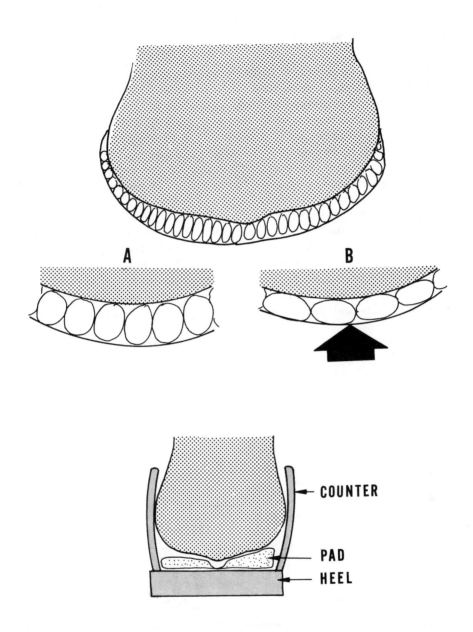

FIGURE 62. Heel padding. *A* reveals the normal heel with the fat lobules contained within connective tissue compartments. In *B* the pressure of the body compresses the lobules and deforms them. In the aged or with trauma, the lobules become filled with a thinner fluid and cannot compress. The septal compartments may also be damaged. The bottom drawing shows the insert for this painful heel. A soft pad with the center hollowed out distributes the pressure around the periphery of the heel.

Chondromalacia Patellae

As the foot goes from heel strike to mid-stance phase, the leg continues to internally rotate causing the foot to pronate. This pronated position finds the foot dorsiflexed, everted, and abducted, all occurring with abrupt force, thus causing some tissues to sustain painful stress.

As the knee flexes 68° in jogging and 85° in running, it is apparent that that difference, combined with the rotation that normally occurs between femur-tibia, the patellofemoral articulation can be stressed, and, therefore, chondromalacia patellae as a complication of sports activities is certainly understandable.

As the knee flexes during mid-stance, the ankle dorsiflexes, being decelerated by the gastroc-soleus muscle group (Fig. 63). A "tight" inflexible gastroc-soleus muscle, erroneously termed "tight heel cord," prevents physiologic heel-knee flexion coordination and the resultant pain can occur from chondromalacia patellae. More knee flexion is needed to cushion the impact that is also cushioned by ankle dorsiflexion. As this latter motion is decreased, more stress is absorbed by the patellofemoral joint.

Plantar Fasciitis

The pronated foot causes plantar fascia stretch normally. However, in the pronated foot, the decreased longitudinal arch plus the trauma of the

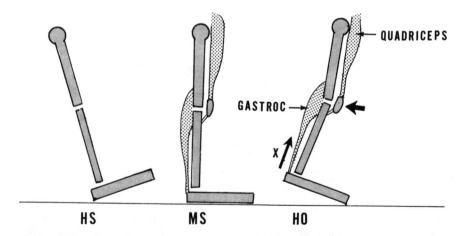

FIGURE 63. Knee stress from a "tight heel cord." HS is heel strike, MS mid-stance, and HO heel-off during gait. At MS the leg proceeds over the planti-foot decelerated by the gastrocnemius as the knee flexes slightly. With a "tight heel cord" this portion of the gait sequence is altered and the knee attempts to flex more to accommodate the lack of ankle motion, thus placing more compression upon the patella with chondromalacia resulting.

70

impact can result in plantar fasciitis. If the stress is excessively forceful or repetitive, the periosteum, to which the plantar fascia attaches, pulls away with resultant hemorrhage subperiostally (Fig. 64). Treatment by heel pads or "cookies" is of no value. Treatment of the pronation is mandatory, as is gentle stretching of the plantar fascia by big toe extension. Injection of steroids into the site of the fasciitis at its site of attachment, originally advocated, has more recently been condemned as causing tissue degeneration and possible fascial tearing.

At toe-off after the heel-off, the leg rotates externally as the foot also supinates. This causes alteration, separation, and approximation of the inferior tibiofibular joint with cortical fracture of the distal fibula. Other stress fractures can occur in the lower tibia, fibula, or both.

Shin Splints

"Shin splints" are an inflammatory condition and can be prevalent in athletic injuries, as the ankle remains dorsiflexed throughout a large phase of running. Shin splints have numerous etiologies. Micro tears may occur at the origin of the anterior or posterior tibialis muscles.

ANTERIOR SHIN SPLINTS. Anterior shin splints may occur during early running, running on hard surfaces, or running down hill when the foot

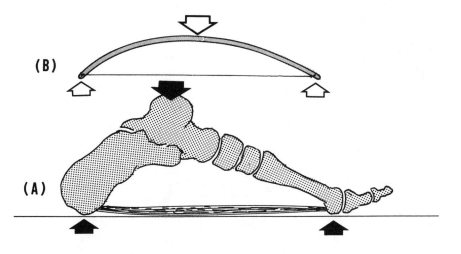

FIGURE 64. Plantar fascia stress during running. A depicts the mechanical stress of weight-bearing (large black arrow) upon the two ground points of contact (small black arrows) with resultant stretch upon the fascia. B depicts the same mechanism upon a stringed bow that is pressed in the direction of the white arrows causing tension upon the string (fascia).

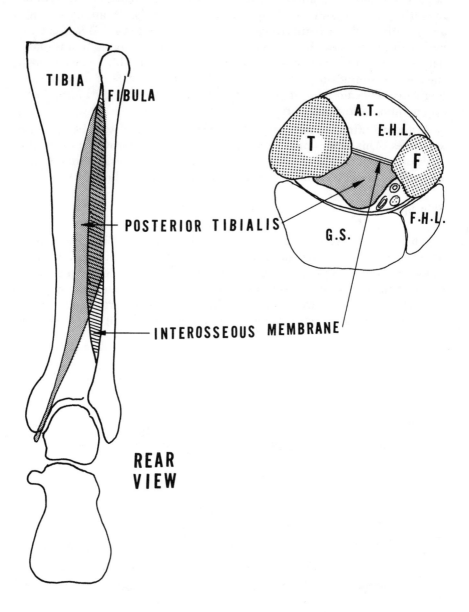

TIBIA

FIBULA

T

A.T.

E.H.L.

F

POSTERIOR TIBIALIS

G.S.

F.H.L.

INTEROSSEOUS MEMBRANE

REAR
VIEW

FIGURE 65. Posterior "shin splint." The posterior tibialis muscle attaches from the interrosseous membrane and the periosteum of the tibia posteriorly. It passes behind the medial malleolus. In a pronated foot or when the posterior tibialis muscle is stressed, microscopic tears can result in its attachment sites causing pain termed "shin splint."

exceeds minimal deceleration after heel strike. A tight heel cord resists elongation of the anterior tibialis and leads to shin splint. Treatment is to rest then stretch the heel cord.

POSTERIOR SHIN SPLINTS. The posterior tibialis muscle irritation causing posterior shin splints occurs in individuals who are moderately to severely pronated, thus placing the posterior muscle on tension stress (Fig. 65). Pain and tenderness are noted at the posterior medial aspect of the tibia where the muscle originates. Treatment here is obviously avoiding hard surfaces for a period, use of taping to supinate the foot, anti-inflammatory drug therapy, and ultimately orthotics to correct the pronation.

Anterior Compartment Syndrome

"Anterior compartment syndrome" is a severe form of anterior shin splint with or without stress fracture. In this syndrome, there is swelling within the tight fascial compartments (Fig. 66). Also, there is severe pain and tenderness that do not respond to rest or icing. Due to compression and ischemia of the anterior tibial nerve, numbness occurs. The extensor hallucis longus muscle becomes affected and weakness results. Ultimate aseptic necrosis, of all the compartment muscle, may occur if fasciec-

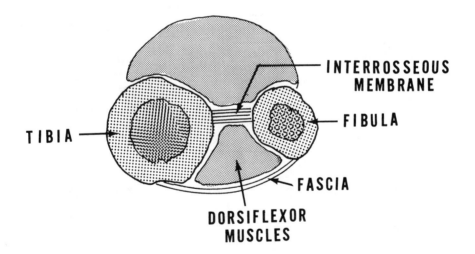

FIGURE 66. Anterior compartment. The anterior compartment of the lower leg which contains the dorsiflexor muscles of the ankle and toes is composed of the tibia and fibula with its connecting interosseous ligament form the posterior wall of the compartment. Anteriorly, there is a firm unyielding fascia that makes the compartment reasonably rigid. Any swelling of the muscle is not accommodated by flexibility of the anterior fascia.

tomy is not performed to decompress the anterior chamber. Ankle sprains of the anterior talofibular ligament may result. These will be discussed in Chapter 10, Injuries to the Ankle.

Peroneal Tendon Dislocation

Peroneal tendon dislocation is a condition resembling, but more severe than, lateral ligamentous sprain. The peroneal tendon passes behind the lateral malleolus and is held there by an overlying retinaculum (Fig. 67). Forceful dorsiflexion with simultaneous peroneal contraction may rupture the retinaculum and dislocate the tendon. Diagnosis is suggested by pain and tenderness at the lateral malleolus and palpating the subluxing tendon. Early diagnosis permits surgical repair of the retinaculum but the tissues atrophy very rapidly and cannot then be repaired. Other corrective surgical procedures are necessary to minimize the pain, dislocation, and instability.

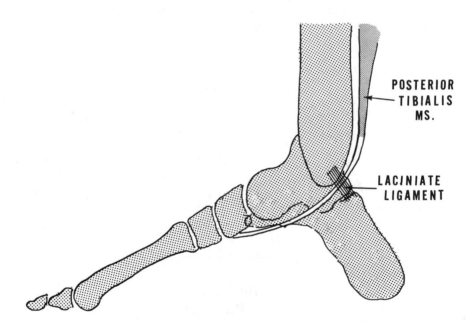

FIGURE 67. The posterior tibial tendon at the medial ankle. The posterior tibial tendon passes under the medial malleolus of the tibia in a tunnel that is covered by the laciniate ligament. In plantar flexion of the foot with inversion, the tendon glides within this compartment. Inflammation of the tendon injury to the laciniate ligament can cause pain at this point or dysfunction of the posterior tibial muscle.

74

Other Conditions

All the conditions of the metatarsal heads, the interdigital neoplasm, and hammer toe can also occur but, other than being aggravated by running or sports, are not unique to these activities. The injuries to the Achilles tendon will be discussed in Chapter 9.

SHOES

Shoes for athletes need specific design for the specific problem. Wide heels supposedly minimize the heel varus-valgus action and decrease knee strain. The rounded heel also decreases impact of heel strike. The counter may be elevated and foam-reinforced to hold the calcaneous snugly. Proper fit and width of the front portion of the shoe avoids stress during anterior shear of athletic activities. Orthotic devices for insertion into shoes must be molded to the foot to insure the proper, desired form of the foot with minimal correction stress.

BIBLIOGRAPHY

COKER, TP, ET AL: *Traumatic lesions of the metatarsophalangeal joint of the great toe in athletes.* Am J Sports Med 326, Nov Dec, 1978.

DEVAS, MB: *Stress fractures of the tibia in athletes or "shin soreness."* J Bone Joint Surg 40B:227, 1958.

DEVAS, MB AND SWEETWAM, R: *Stress fractures of the fibula: A review of fifty cases in athletics.* J Bone Joint Surg 30B:818, 1956.

DISTEFANO, V AND NIXON, JE: *An improved method of taping.* Am J Sports Med 2:209, 1974.

JONES, E: *Operative treatment of chronic dislocations of the peroneal tendons.* J Bone Joint Surg 14:574, 1932.

KENNEDY, JC AND WILLIS, RB: *The effects of local steroid injections in tendons: A biomechanical and microscopic correlative study.* Am J Sports Med 4:11, 1976.

KULAND, DN: *The foot in athletics.* In HELFET, AJ AND LEE, DM (EDS): *Disorders of the Foot.* JB Lippincott, Philadelphia, 1980, pp 59-79.

SARMIENTO, A AND WOLF, M: *Subluxation of peroneal tendons: Case treated by rerouting tendons under calcaneo fibular ligament.* J Bone Joint Surg 57A:115, 1970.

SLOCUM, DB: *Overuse syndromes of the lower leg and foot in the athletes.* AAOS Instructional Course Lectures 17:359, 1960.

SLOCUM, DB AND BOWERMAN, W: *The biomechanics of running.* Clin Orthop 23:39, 1962.

STOVER, CN AND BRYAN, DR: *Traumatic dislocation of the peroneal tendons.* Am J Surg 103:180, 1962.

CHAPTER 5

The Foot in Childhood

Many common foot problems seen at birth and during early childhood, if recognized and treated early, may respond to conservative treatment. Such abnormalities are more common than the literature indicates. In most cases, the causative factors are more conjectural than scientific but if the mechanism causing the abnormality is recognized, appropriate corrective treatment may cure or at least minimize the deformity.

CLASSIFICATION OF FOOT DEFORMITIES

Foot deformities are generally classified into four positions: (1) *equinus* in which the heel is elevated and the foot is plantar flexed, (2) *calcaneus* in which the foot is dorsiflexed and the heel relatively depressed, (3) *varus** in which the foot is inverted and adducted, and (4) *valgus** in

---

*There is considerable confusion in the terminology used to describe position and movement of the foot.

Varus implies that the distal member of an extremity is bent *toward* the midline. The apex of the angle formed by the longitudinal axes of the component bones points away from the midline. The heel is rotated inward on its longitudinal axis or is inverted (Gartland).

Valgus means bent or turned *from* the midline. The apex of the angle formed by the longitudinal axes of the component bones points *toward* the midline. The heel in valgus is everted or rotated outward on its longitudinal axis (Gartland).

Movement about an axis passing transversely through the foot is *dorsiflexion-plantar flexion*. Movement about a vertical axis is *abduction-adduction* and about a longitudinal axis *inversion-eversion*.

Inversion implies elevation of the inner border of the foot and *eversion* elevation of the outer border. Adduction-abduction occurs chiefly at the tarsometatarsal joints. Inversion and adduction combine to constitute *supination* and also varus of the forefoot, whereas eversion and abduction cause *pronation* or valgus of the foot.

MacConaill views the foot as a "twisted osteo-fibrous plate" by which the intrauterine position of the lower limb is in pronation and any lessening of the foot torsion is supination. The foot is thus supinated when it has been "untwisted."

which the foot assumes a position of eversion and abduction. Deformities may consist of just one of the above positions, but the majority are combinations in which equinus is associated with varus or valgus, or calcaneus with varus or valgus (Fig. 68).

ETIOLOGIC CONCEPTS

The majority of foot deformities noted in infants are flatfoot and equinovarus deformities. Valgus, varus, equinus, and calcaneus abnormalities comprise the remainder. These abnormalities are considered to be congenital, acquired, or a residual of neurologic abnormalities.

Delay or arrested derotation of the intrauterine position is one of the intriguing concepts of the causation of the abnormal foot. About the third month of intrauterine existence the fetus has its thighs flexed, abducted, and outwardly rotated with its legs crossed. The feet are plantar flexed and adducted with the plantar surfaces held against its own abdomen (Fig. 69). As the fetus develops, the thighs derotate inwardly and the feet gradually turn out to become placed against the uterine wall. If, for some reason, derotation of the feet is arrested, the child is born with the feet still plantar flexed and inverted in the equinovarus position.

Internal Tibial Torsion

There is 30° of internal tibial torsion at birth which becomes neutral at age 2 and 15° of external rotation by age 3. Infants' legs are naturally bowed, becoming straight by 18 to 20 months, becoming knock-kneed by 30 months and remaining knock-kneed by age 6 to 7. With the normal variation, it is obvious that treatment must be precisely evaluated as natural evolution may indicate therapeutic success rather than natural correction that would have occurred without treatment. Patient reassurance and periodic evaluation is, therefore, indicated.

The foot as a source of deformity rather than tibial or femoral malalignment must be determined. Metabolic bone disease, abnormal epiphyseal growth, and congenital or post-traumatic conditions must be ruled out if severe or persistent deformity exists.

Faulty sleeping habits are blamed for persistence of leg deformity (see Fig. 69), but this is not verified. In 18-month-old children, correction of the persistent internal tibial torsion may be treated by use of a Denis Browne night splint (Fig. 70), but this is poorly tolerated by children in later years (i.e., age 3 or older). Gradually rotating the shoes within the Denis Browne type of splint is gained from the initial 0 to 20° of internal rotation. Further rotation places stress upon the knees. To be of value, the splint must be worn 12 hours daily. One year of wearing usually accomplishes its purpose. As stated later, with severe metatarsus varus and inter-

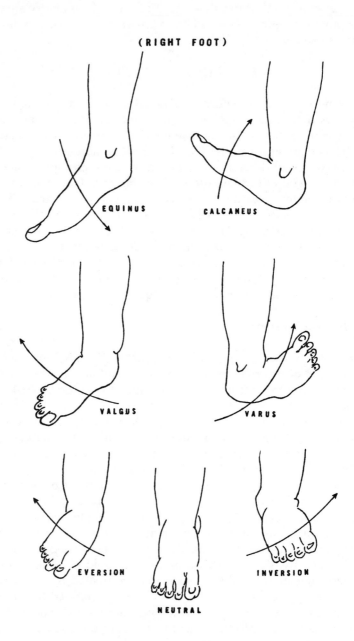

FIGURE 68. Terminology of foot abnormalities or positions.

78

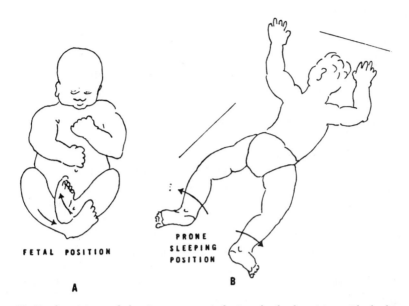

FIGURE 69. Fetal position and sleeping posture. A depicts the fetal position with the hips flexed, abducted, and rotated outwardly. The feet are usually plantar flexed and adducted with plantar surface against the abdomen. The sleeping position (B) will maintain the newborn position. In this illustration both feet are abducted. The foot position varies with the immeduate postpartum position.

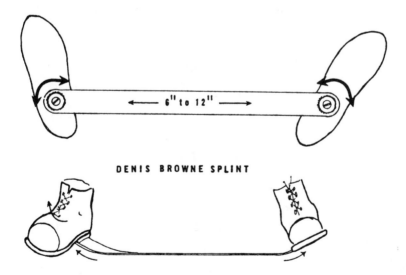

FIGURE 70. The Denis Browne splint. The spreader bar, which may be metal, plastic, or wood is firmly attached to a pair of shoes. The shoe attachment may be fixed or adjustable so that the shoes can be turned in or out, everted or inverted, as the need dictates. The width of the spreader bar depends on the desired abduction of the legs and hips.

nal tibial torsion, the splint may be justifiably applied at an earlier stage in life.

"Cable Twisters" (see Fig. 78 later in this chapter) have been advocated by some for treatment of internal tibial torsion but this has not been verified and results have been disappointing.

Bowlegs

Outward bowing of the tibia can be considered normal in children up to age 20 to 24 months. This condition is frequently associated with internal tibial torsion. Treatment is usually not indicated unless the associated internal tibial torsion is severe and persistent, then treatment is directed to the torsion rather than to the bowing. Denis Browne splints are contraindicated in treating the combination of bowing *and* internal rotation, as the splint places stress upon the medial ligaments of the knee and accentuates the ultimate knock-knee that can then evolve. Unilateral bowing should alert the physician of the possibility of bone dysplasia, neurofibromatosis, or Blount's disease (tibia varus).

CENTERS OF OSSIFICATION

At birth, the foot consists of as much soft tissue as bone. X-ray examination of the foot shows only the diaphysis of the phalanges and the metatarsals and the nuclei of the calcaneus and talus (Fig. 71). Only the calca-

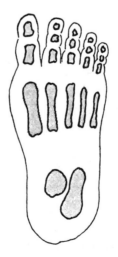

FIGURE 71. X-ray film of foot in the newborn. In the newborn only the diaphyses of the phalanges and metatarsals along with the nuclei of the talus and calcaneus are visible.

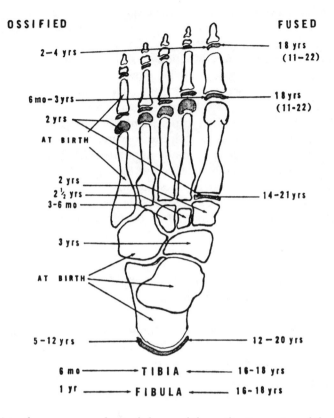

OSSIFIED   FUSED

2–4 yrs   18 yrs (11–22)

6 mo–3 yrs   18 yrs (11–22)

2 yrs

AT BIRTH

2 yrs
2½ yrs   14–21 yrs
3–6 mo

3 yrs

AT BIRTH

5–12 yrs   12–20 yrs

6 mo ⟶ TIBIA ⟵ 16–18 yrs

1 yr ⟶ FIBULA ⟵ 16–18 yrs

FIGURE 72. Age of appearance and age of closure of the ossification centers of the foot.

neus, talus, and occasionally the cuboid are ossified at birth; the remainder of the bones are still cartilage. Growth continues from infancy through adolescence and Figure 72 shows the ages at which the centers of ossification appear and fuse. During this period of growth, structural changes in the foot may be caused by abnormal stresses. By the time it is full-grown, the foot is 90 percent bone.

FOOT POSTURES OF THE NEWBORN

The conditions of equinus or calcaneus with either varus or valgus should be recognized early. Manual testing will determine whether the foot is sufficiently flexible to permit correction of the deformity. If the foot is flexible enough and the deformity easily altered, stretching of the soft tissues is begun immediately. The abnormality is demonstrated to the parents, and the tissue-stretching exercises taught so the child can receive the stretching several times a day. The specific exercises must be carefully prescribed, explained, and demonstrated to the parents and their performance observed for accuracy.

The forefoot may be in adduction or abduction and in mild supination or pronation. The forefoot can be moved in either direction with the other hand holding the calcaneus firmly. This maneuver tests the flexibility of the forefoot and also becomes a manner of treating any existing inflexibility. Once established as pertinent, the movement is taught to the parents. If a tight Achilles tendon is discovered, this too can be stretched by the parents. They must be made aware that elevation of the forefoot does not necessarily stretch the Achilles tendon (see Fig. 32). Only when the calcaneus is "pulled down" does the heel cord get stretched. The foot that is pronated (everted) usually has a shortened Achilles tendon, and to be stretched properly the foot must be inverted during the stretching exercises.

The calcaneus deformity (see Fig. 68) may reveal contracture of the dorsiflexors and the toe extensors. These can be stretched by grasping the leg and gradually, firmly, and repeatedly forcing the foot into plantar flexion. The toes can be flexed simultaneously thus stretching the toe extensors.

If the deformed foot does not become more flexible and appear more nearly normal after four to six weeks of daily passive stretching, mechanical devices are indicated. Because soft-tissue changes cause and maintain the foot deformity, gradual stretching of the foot into a more physiologic position can be achieved by plaster casting or by bracing. The attempt is always made to *overcorrect* the deformity so that when the tissues are released, they will return with the foot to the normal position and not a partially deformed posture. Plaster casting is more satisfactory than bracing because it is skintight and by proper molding can correct the specific portion of the foot desired. Also, plaster is obviously less expensive than bracing.

The newly acquired position of overcorrection is held for one to four weeks by maintaining the cast or by bivalving the cast and applying it for varying portions of the day with interspersed exercises. Exercises must be resumed when the cast is ultimately removed. If the foot is large enough to be fitted with a "corrective" shoe, the correction can thus be maintained. The term "corrective" is questioned because no shoe corrects a deformity; it merely holds the correction gained by other means.

Knock-Knees

Knock-knees, medically termed genu valgum, is noted in most children to some degree up to age 20 months. It generally self-corrects by age 6 to 7. It appears to be at its worst angulation at the age of 5.

82

Severe knock-knees may benefit from a night splint or a night brace, but this is rarely needed, and surgery is only considered when there is a separation of the feet and ankles of 8 to 10 inches. This severe deformity casess little foot deformity, but does cause an awkward gait, knee pain, and subluxation of the patella.

Along with knock-knees, these children also have flat feet and some "toeing out." As an unsightly gait is the major manifestation, an inner heel wedge with a longitudinal pad will improve the gait. However, there is no scientific documentation that it corrects the genu valgum or the pronated feet.

Femoral Anteversion

This is internal rotation of the hip, which is the major cause of "toeing in" in children. Anteversion (see Fig. 68) is in the vicinity of 45° at birth, then gradually decreases to become 15° at age 8. If excessive anteversion persists, there are physiologic attempts at corrections by external tibial torsion. If there is simultaneous internal torsion, toeing in, therefore, becomes marked.

Although improper sitting or lying positions (see Fig. 69) have been implicated and correcting these positions has been advocated, this has not been scientifically proven beneficial. Normal evolutionary correction is expected and learned muscular control and gait training are gradually rewarding. The progress requires dynamic exercises to externally rotate the hips and participation in sports or activities that encourage this normal movement. This includes roller skating, ice skating, ballet, and gymnastic exercises. Shoe corrections to evert the foot have been advocated. This consists of an outer heel wedge, (1/8″), an outer sole wedge, (1/8″), and a navicular pad (3/16″) under the arch. The twister cable brace may be worn at night, but not for daily walking use.

Surgery is rarely indicated, but in severe disabling conditions an osteotomy with decreased internal rotation of the femur is possible and can be advocated.

Flatfoot

At birth, all infants' feet appear flat, that is, without a longitudinal arch. This is due to excessive fat in the arch and this condition resolves itself usually during the first 18 months. Children with a flexible flatfoot may have a tight heel that aggravates the symptomatic flexible foot.

The excessive flexible foot presents a common variety of flatfoot in children. This is due to ligamentous laxity in which the foot has an apparent arch when not weight bearing, but completely flattens during weight bearing. Manual examination reveals excessive mobility of all the joints in

83

the foot. As excessive flatfoot may be caused by a vertical talus, a tarsal coalition, or cerebral palsy, this must be kept in mind during the examination and verified by x-ray examination.

Treatment, of the excessively flexible flatfoot, is usually not necessary unless the child is symptomatic, that is, complains of leg cramps that simulate shin splints. The child may walk with a toe-in gait, in spite of no internal femoral torsion, to avoid symptomatic pronation. The child may also develop painful calluses over the medial aspect of the foot. Treatment includes an inner heel wedge of $1/16$ to $1/8$ of an inch. The Thomas heel should be used only in a child who does not walk with an inverted gait, that is, a toe-in gait. Otherwise, an awkward gait is encouraged. A firm longitudinal arch support and rigid shoes may be uncomfortable and have no corrective value.

Congenital Flatfoot

The congenital foatfoot is relatively rare but when present is more severe than the acquired flatfoot (Fig. 73). In the flexible congenital flatfoot, the position is one of calcaneovalgus with the foot folded laterally upon itself. It can be brought downward with relative ease and can be so maintained until muscular action and weight bearing develop. It is maintained by daily exercising and a shoe that holds the foot in the corrected position or a plaster cast that is bivalved and worn for varying periods.

Rigid Flatfoot

The rigid flatfoot is more difficult to treat. In this condition the heel is firmly held in a marked valgus position and the forefoot in marked eversion. There is almost a reversal of the longitudinal arch which appears convex rather than concave and bulges at its midpoint. X-ray examination reveals that the talus faces medially and downward, and the navicular rests on the superior surface of the neck of the talus rather than in front of its head. Correction of this condition requires a series of plaster casts to change the convexity of the arch and to return the navicular to its normal place. Surgery is frequently needed to accomplish this but, with either method of treatment, the results are frequently disappointing and surgical arthrodesis is required in later life if the foot becomes painful.

Acquired Flatfoot

The acquired flatfoot is usually flexible and may appear well formed when not weight bearing or when standing on tiptoes. The foot pronates when weight bearing and assumes a flattened appearance. The longitudinal arch becomes effaced, the navicular depresses toward the floor, and

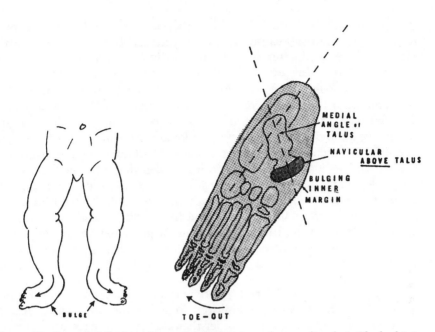

FIGURE 73. Congenital flatfoot. Congenital flatfoot is a calcaneovalgus foot. The heel is in valgus and the talus points medially toward the other foot forming an angle with the calcaneus. The talus points *downward* rather than forward and the navicular lies on the superior surface of the neck of the talus instead of anterior to the head.

the calcaneus undergoes eversion. The medial border loses its concavity and actually appears to bulge. If the flatfoot is mobile, it regains much of its longitudinal arch upon arising on tiptoes.

A child with pronated feet develops an awkward gait. The child walks "toeing out" and lacks "spring" in the gait. Later, there may be complaints of aching in the calf and leg muscles. It is this complaint or the parental concern over the awkward gait that brings them to the doctor.

Pronation may be associated with generalized ligamentous laxity, in which case the child also has excessive mobility in the hips, knees, elbows, and low back. This patient is often referred to as "double-jointed" as an expression of hyperextensibility. Hypoflexibility may also cause pronation when tightness of the Achilles tendon causes pronation of the foot to permit full weight bearing. Discovery of a tight Achilles tendon during the examination reveals the cause of the pronation.

Internal Tibial Torsion

Moderate to severe internal tibial torsion may cause the foot to evert in weight bearing to compensate the torsion and allow the foot to face straight ahead. The "toe-in" stance is partially corrected by the eversion of the forefoot but this causes the foot to pronate. Internal rotation of the tibia rarely persists after infancy. It is estimated that only 10 percent of children reaching age 5 have residual internal tibial torsion, and less than 5 percent continue to have rotation into adolescence. Since internal rotation of the legs, especially internal tibial torsion, is usually gone by adulthood, no treatment is necessary other than elimination and avoidance of obvious postural and positional factors in the newborn state.

Pronation can be acquired after prolonged bed rest or immobilization of the foot and leg in a plaster cast, but it has been claimed to be the result of faulty sleeping habits during the first four months of life. When children sleep prone with the legs in a frog position (see Fig. 69B), the hips flexed, abducted, and externally rotated. The firm mattress and bulky diapers encourage this posture. In this position all the pressure is imposed upon the inner border of the foot causing pronation. The foot invertors are thus stretched and the evertors permitted to shorten. The mechanism of pronation is instituted.

The external rotators of the hips are normally stronger than the internal rotators and this encourages children to sit on the floor with the hips externally rotated and the feet under them. There is a tendency, however, to sit in this position with the feet turned outward, and the floor pressure against the inner border of the feet tends to pronate them.

TREATMENT OF THE PRONATED FOOT

Positioning

Treatment of the pronated foot must be considered before the child walks and be continued when walking begins. Pre-walking treatment consists of altering the faulty sleeping posture, gaining and maintaining flexibility of internal rotation of the entire leg, and exercising the foot to acquire an inverted supinated foot with a longitudinal arch. Specific ways of doing these must be carefully outlined to the parents.

If the newborn child cannot be forced to sleep on the back without danger of regurgitation of food and aspiration, it may be possible to cause the child to sleep on the side by propping with pillows. Frequent observation during the night and nap time are obviously required to maintain this position. Thick and multiple diapers must be avoided to minimize the frog position.

If the external rotators of the hip are tight, they should be stretched many times daily by the parent. This is done with the child lying on the back with the legs extended. The parent grasps the lower thighs, rotates both legs inwardly as far as they will go, and holds them in this position for 30 to 40 seconds. This exercise should be repeated several times daily and the parent must be instructed that *stretching is the intention*. Each exercise should attempt further internal rotation until flexibility is achieved.

Exercises

The foot must be exercised to force it into adduction and supination to form a longitudinal arch. The parents must be taught how to stretch the foot and advised to do it frequently and patiently. After each stretching treatment, the foot should be held in the newly acquired position for 30 to 45 seconds which insures that the foot will remain flexible. This period is arbitrary but gives the parents a time factor as a goal. Figure 74 demonstrates the maneuver required to form the longitudinal arch. An adult foot has been used in the illustration for clarity. In treating the child's foot, the hand positions may need to be altered to fit the smaller foot, but the principles remain the same.

The child with pronated feet frequently walks awkwardly, toeing-out and with no "spring" in the gait. Later in life this child frequently develops aching in the legs and curtails activities which causes greater pronation as a result of disuse and deconditioning.

The child who exhibits tibial torsion may stand with the feet pronated although the walk has a toe-in gait. The stance with the foot facing

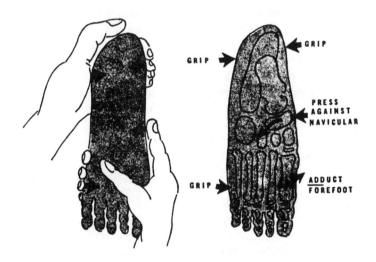

FIGURE 74. Forming an arch in a flatfoot by stretching. Illustration depicts the technique of stretching the right foot. The heel is gripped by the *left* hand holding the calcaneus in a neutral position. The index finger of the *right* hand presses against the navicular bone while the fingers of the *right* hand adduct the forefoot around the fulcrum of the index finger pressing the navicular area. For the left foot the procedure is reversed. In the illustration the right foot is viewed from above.

87

straight ahead is done by everting and pronating the foot. The toe-in gait permits the child to bear weight on the lateral border of the foot and causes the foot to supinate and form a longitudinal arch. Toe-in gait in this condition *should be encouraged* and not discouraged or corrected. This compensatory gait occurs naturally and strengthens the foot, improves the arch, and ultimately leads to a good painless gait. The tendency to place lateral wedges on the sole and heel of the shoes to correct the toeing-in *should be discouraged* as this merely enhances pronation of the foot.

Treatment of the pronated foot must provide support for the longitudinal arch and must attempt to cause supination. The obese phlegmatic child should be made to lose weight and be encouraged to exercise. Proper walking is the best exercise for this patient, and the tendency to avoid walking must not be allowed.

Shoe Corrections

For the newborn, no shoes are indicated and when there is an abnormality present, no shoe is "corrective." Correction consists of exercise, plaster casts, or even braces. A shoe can only maintain a correction, once flexibility has been gained, and assist in improving the gait.

The normal foot should be fitted with a blucher type shoe having a broad toe, lacing across a tongue, and preferably a low quarter (see Fig. 29). A high-top shoe offers no support and does not "strengthen" the foot or the ankle. If correction is sought, the shoe last must be formed in the manner and direction desired. In the pronated foot, the sole of the shoe, the *last*, should turn in, and the counter should grip the heel in a snug fit. Any correction incorporated into the shoe will be ineffectual if the heel is free to move about the counter (Fig. 75). Pronation may also be partially corrected by elevating the inner side of the heel $1/16$ to $3/16$ of an inch. The exact elevation will depend upon the severity of the heel valgus (Fig. 76). A Thomas heel is frequently prescribed to carry the medial counter forward and give a more anterior pivot point to help supinate the foot during walking.

The shank of the shoe should not be too firm or inflexible. A completely inflexible shank prevents normal use of the intrinsic muscles of the foot and defeats the purpose of any correction. A high-top shoe has merely the advantage of being difficult for the child to remove.

Supports

If pronation is severe and the longitudinal arch totally depressed but the foot is flexible, an arch support may be considered. The supports are molded over a plaster mold of the foot to conform to the exact contour

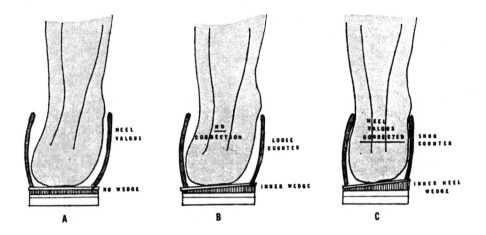

FIGURE 75. Necessity of snug heel in correcting heel valgus. *A* shows a valgus heel within a regular shoe. *B* shows that an inner wedge in the heel of a loose-fitting shoe does *not* correct the valgus. To be effective an inner wedge has to be placed on a shoe counter that "hugs" the heel *(C)*.

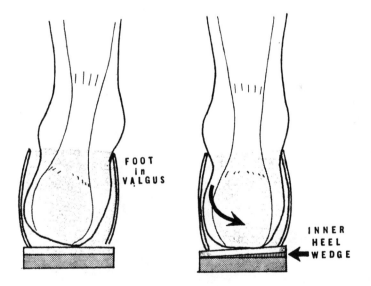

FIGURE 76. Inner heel wedge in treatment of heel valgus. The inner wedge should taper from no elevation at the outer border to $1/16$ to $3/16$ of an inch on the inner border. The exact elevation is determined by the height needed to place the calcaneus in a near-vertical position.

89

desired for the specific foot. Made of felt or sponge rubber covered with leather, the supports tend to deform or compress under the weight of the patient and must be replaced frequently. A rigid arch may be made of metal or plastic, but it frequently causes pressure discomfort. The longitudinal arch support must elevate the arch with its apex under the navicular. The support must extend forward to end behind the first three metatarsal heads, must taper laterally to present no elevation under the lateral border of the foot, and must extend backward to end just anterior to the calcaneal weight-bearing edge. It must form the contour of a symmetrical arch and be comfortable.

A plastic arch support, based upon the principle that the weight-bearing foot *supinates* when the leg rotates externally (see Fig. 60) and forms a longitudinal arch, has been designed by the Biomechanics Laboratory of the University of California. A mold of the foot is made from a plastic plaster applied skintight over a thin rubber covering. The foot is then placed on a rotating platform and the leg, with the foot weight-bearing, is externally rotated. The mold hardens in this supinated position. Using a positive cast made from the mold, the arch support is made of a fiber glass material. The support fits the heel snugly, thus maintaining the acquired vertical position of the calcaneus, and the forefoot is held in supination by the medial and lateral phalanges (Fig. 77). This technique is not yet

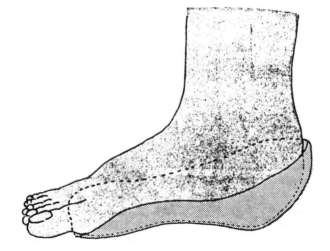

FIGURE 77. The UC-BL shoe insert. The laminated fiber glass insert shell is molded over a plaster mold of the foot. It fits snugly into the shoe. The heel is held in a neutral position and the forefoot held in an adducted supinated position.

90

known by many orthotists and may be difficult to procure, but it is based on sound physiologic principles and should ultimately receive wide acceptance.

Gait Training

Exercise is the most beneficial form of treatment of the pronated foot. Corrective shoes and arch supports are essentially "crutches" to be considered as a means to an end and not ends in themselves. The exercises must be modified according to the child's age and ability to cooperate. The heel cord must be sufficiently extensible to permit more than 90° of dorsiflexion (see Fig. 41). The gastroc-soleus group must be strong and can be strengthened by exercises such as rising on the toes or walking on tiptoes.

The intrinsic muscles of the foot can be strengthened by toe-flexor exercises such as picking up marbles, wrinkling a towel lying on the floor, or standing on the outer border of both feet and actively flexing the toes while in this position.

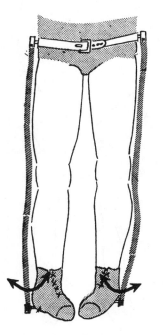

FIGURE 78. Orthotic "twisters" to control internal or external rotation. The "twisters" are coiled springs within a cable housing that resists torque. By its attachment at the pelvic band and to the shoe the foot can be made to turn *in* or *out* by adjustment. It permits ambulation and controls the rotation in both the stance and swing phases of walking.

Teaching a child to walk with a heel-toe gait and the feet turned out about 10° may, by constant repetition, result in the child adopting this method as the subconscious manner of walking. In the very severe case, where toeing-in (or toeing-out) cannot be voluntarily controlled or exists in a child too young to cooperate, "twisters" (Fig. 78) may be used.

Toe-in gait, commonly called "pigeon-toed," may result from excessive anteversion of the femoral neck (see Fig. 36), congenital hip dislocation, knock-knee, marked internal tibial torsion, or metatarsus varus. The exact patho-mechanics of the gait must be discovered and, if possible, be corrected.

METATARSUS VARUS

Metatarsus varus is a common condition in newborns (Fig. 79). It is also termed metatarsus adductus and some would differentiate the two terms, but they are sufficiently similar to use the names interchangeably.

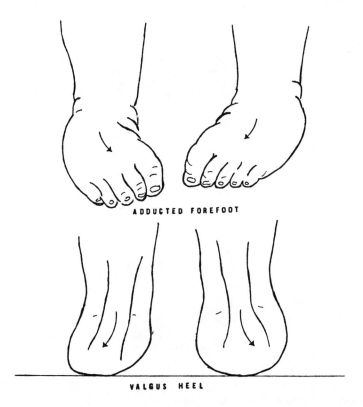

ADDUCTED FOREFOOT

VALGUS HEEL

FIGURE 79. Metatarsus varus. The foot in metatarsus varus has an adducted forefoot, a convex lateral foot border, and the heel is in valgus. No equinus is present.

Diagnosis

Metatarsus varus is not a severe deformity but children may walk in an awkward manner, have a toe-in gait, and frequently "trip" over their own feet. They wear out shoes early and distort them. This condition may be adequately corrected but recurrences are frequent, and correction without adequate and prolonged follow-up leads to failure.

The following components of metatarsus varus (Fig. 80) must be recognized to establish proper diagnosis and to ensure adequate treatment: (1) the anterior segment of the foot is in *adduction*, (2) the lateral border of the foot is convex with the apex of the convexity appearing at the base of the fifth metatarsal, (3) the heel is in *valgus*, (4) internal tibial torsion is frequently present, (5) there is a sharp angulation of the medial border of the foot at the tarsometatarsal joint, (6) the first metatarsal is more angu-

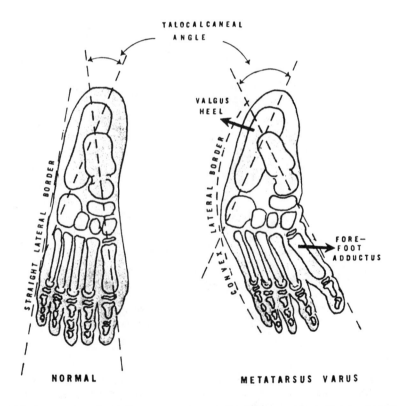

FIGURE 80. Components of metatarsus varus compared to the normal foot. Metatarsus varus has an adducted forefoot and a valgus heel. The lateral margin of the foot is convex with the apex at the base of the fifth metatarsal. The talus is medially and anteriorly displaced in relationship to the calcaneus thus increasing the talo calcaneal angle.

lated than the other four but all are angulated, (7) the talus is medially and anteriorly displaced in its relation to the calcaneus, and (8) there is no equinus and no limitation of dorsiflexion as is seen in talipes equinovarus or "clubfoot."

Treatment

Treatment should be instituted early. In many cases the condition corrects itself in time, but the large percentage of cases in which it persists and causes cosmetic and slight functional impairment justifies early vigorous treatment. Exercises administered by the parents are usually ineffectual. A Denis Browne splint has the danger of everting the feet thus accentuating the heel valgus without correcting the forefoot. Reversing the shoes by putting the right on the left foot and vice versa may hold the

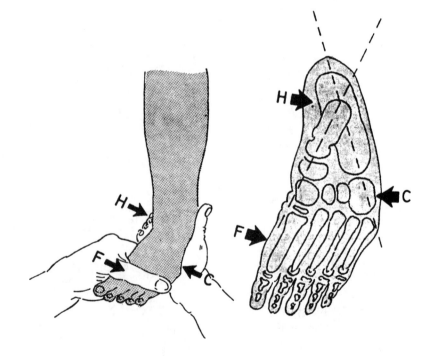

FIGURE 81. Technique of manipulating metatarsus varus. Illustration shows the method of correcting metatarsus varus during plaster casting. Pressure (C) against the cuboid and anterior portion of the calcaneus medially forces the calcaneus under the talus and thus corrects the valgus. H is traction on the posterior aspect of the calcaneus to aid C in moving the calcaneus into a neutral or varus position. F is simultaneous pressure by the other hand to correct the adducted metatarsals. All pressures are applied simultaneously.

94

mild flexible metatarsus varus in a corrected position but does not correct the moderate or severe adductus. A series of plaster casts that simultaneously correct the forefoot and the hindfoot have been found effective. The heel is forced medially, the calcaneus moves under the talus, and the heel is placed into the varus position. This maneuver requires pressure upon the cuboid while moving the calcaneus, and the forefoot is simultaneously forced into abduction (Fig. 81). Pronation of the forefoot must be avoided. Before the cast is permitted to dry fully, the transverse metatarsal arch can be molded into slight dorsal convexity (see Fig. 12). Each cast should be left on for two weeks before it is replaced by a cast that attempts further correction. Casting is continued until the foot is slightly *overcorrected.*

The cast is applied with the foot in slight equinus and in slight inversion to the long axis of the leg. The toes should be left exposed. The position of the heel is better controlled if the cast extends above the knee which also permits external rotation of the leg to correct any associated internal tibial torsion.

Metatarsus varus must not be confused with talipes equinovarus ("clubfoot"). In metatarsus varus the heel is in the valgus position, whereas in talipes equinovarus it is in varus. The clubfoot is in equinus and resists dorsiflexion due to contracted posterior leg muscles. The metatarsus varus has free dorsiflexion and the foot can be dorsiflexed sufficiently to bring the dorsum of the foot in contact with the tibia. In the metatarsus varus foot the calcaneus can usually be moved easily into the varus position, whereas in clubfoot the heel is "fixed" in the varus position.

METATARSUS PRIMUS VARUS

Diagnosis

Metatarsus primus varus is a condition that mimics metatarsus varus but only the first metatarsal is in adduction and all the other metatarsals are in proper alignment. The first metatarsal is angulated medially upon the medial cuneiform or may be aligned to a deformed cuneiform (Fig. 82). The lateral border of the foot does not show the convexity noted in metatarsus varus. Treatment is usually unnecessary.

TALIPES EQUINOVARUS (CONGENITAL CLUBFOOT)

Talipes equinovarus, commonly termed "clubfoot," is considered the most significant congenital fixed deformity of the foot. Found more commonly in boys than in girls, it is considered a defect in prenatal development and may occur in one or both feet.

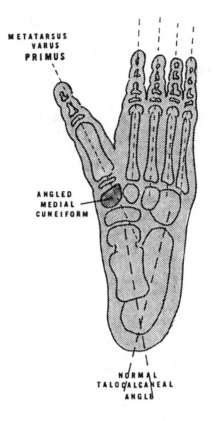

METATARSUS
VARUS
PRIMUS

ANGLED
MEDIAL
CUNEIFORM

NORMAL
TALOCALCANEAL
ANGLE

FIGURE 82. Metatarsus primus varus. Primus varus grossly resembles metatarsus varus but in primus only the first metatarsal is in adduction. The remaining metatarsals are in proper alignment. The first metatarsal may adduct because of a deformed medial cuneiform or may be angled medially upon a normal cuneiform. The talocalcaneal angle reveals no deviation of the talar relationship upon the calcaneus.

Diagnosis

The condition is characterized by the following components: (1) inversion *(twisting inward)* and adduction *(inward deviation)* of the forefoot (Fig. 83), (2) varus of the calcaneus *(inversion of the heel)*, (3) equinus *(plantar flexion)*, (4) contraction of the tissues on the medial side of the foot, (5) underdeveloped evertor muscles on the lateral side of the leg, (6) underdeveloped and contracted calf muscles, and (7) resistance to passive correction.

A plantar flexed inverted foot in the newborn that cannot be brought into a dorsiflexed or everted position suggests talipes equinovarus. This is

96

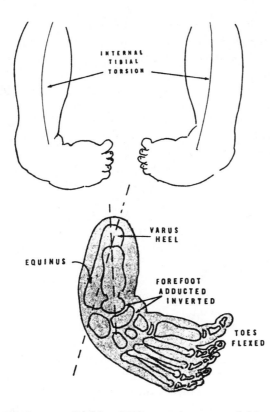

FIGURE 83. Talipes equinovarus: "clubfoot." Talipes equinovarus or clubfoot has an inflexible adducted forefoot and a varus heel. The toes are usually flexed. The medial tissues of the foot and ankle are contracted, the Achilles tendon is shortened, and there is usually some internal tibial torsion. These deformities resist passive stretching.

contrary to the normal child's foot, which may be plantar flexed and inverted but is completely flexible. It differs from the metatarsus varus foot in which the heel is in valgus and mobile. In clubfoot, the toes also are flexed and resist extension and there is usually an associated internal tibial torsion. The child stands bearing weight on the base of the fifth metatarsal bone.

Treatment

Treatment must be instituted immediately after birth by corrective plaster casting. Time is of the essence and procrastination by instituting ineffectual massage, corrective shoes, and passive exercises only delays proper treatment and decreases the probability of correction.

Prognosis relative to the degree of improvement is guarded, as the tissues creating the deformity are atrophic, fibrosed, and contracted. There is also an irreversible muscular imbalance. Treatment aims to prevent bony and articular deformity and to minimize fibrous contracture. Recurrence is possible even after adequate correction in early childhood, thus a long-term program of observation and treatment must be instituted. The initial treatment is to correct, then to overcorrect, and maintain the corrected position of the foot until bone structure is fully developed. Recurrence then is less likely to occur.

Casts applied to the newborn are changed at each stage of correction. If the child is over 2 months of age, the initial casts can safely be wedged. The cast should be applied to the foot covered with a thin layer of Webril or felt so that the contours can be molded yet the bony prominences protected. Correction is made by firm manual pressure *correcting the adductus* and *inversion first* and making *no attempt to alter the equinus.* The cast should be molded carefully and should not be modified once the plaster has begun to set. Alteration after partial drying may cause wrinkling of the cast, forming pressure points against vulnerable areas of the foot. A faulty or unsatisfactory cast should be removed and reapplied.

Attempting correction of equinus concurrently with correction of the adductus and inversion may result in the formation of a "rocker bottom." "Rocker bottom" implies reversal of the longitudinal arch with a convex rather than concave plantar surface. The equinus calf contracture resists elongation, and efforts to correct the equinus initially may cause dorsiflexion of the forefoot upon the hind foot and reverses the longitudinal arch.

Casts are applied and changed once or twice a week, first correcting the adducted forefoot and ultimately achieving overcorrection. The calcaneus is brought under the talus and the heel placed in the valgus position. The cast is extended to include the flexed knee which controls the position sought for the heel.

The contracted Achilles tendon becomes more resistant to elongation by this delay, but the forefoot must be corrected to prevent recurrence and to minimize the formation of a rocker bottom. Once the adductus and inversion are overcorrected, the equinus is gradually corrected by progressive dorsiflexion of the ankle.

Internal tibial torsion may be corrected by externally rotating the leg since the plaster cast extends to include the flexed knee. A Denis Browne type of splint may be incorporated into the plaster casts of the feet to gain external rotation and abduction, but the use of a Denis Browne splint without plaster casting the feet will not correct the major deformities of the heel and forefoot.

The foot once corrected can be maintained in this acquired position by bivalved plaster casts or by corrective shoes externally rotated on a Denis

Browne bar (see Fig. 70). Surgical correction is indicated if correction has not been achieved within four months by casting. There currently is a tendency to operate earlier to re-establish the normal relationship of the tarsal bones and to remove the deforming forces of muscles and soft tissues. Instances of recurrence are claimed to be less with early surgical intervention, but as yet conclusive evidence is lacking.

Operative procedures involve the following: (1) soft tissue release of medial border tissues and lengthening of the Achilles tendon, (2) tendon transplants to change evertors to invertors and dorsiflexors (The anterior tibial tendon, which is basically an invertor-dorsiflexor, is transferred laterally to the base of the third metatarsal to become an evertor. The posterior tibial tendon, a powerful plantar flexor-invertor, is released or is transferred laterally.), and (3) osteotomy or arthrodesis in which the bones and their joints are remolded and fused in the newly acquired position. In later life, triple arthrodesis may be necessary to reform the foot. Detailed discussion of operative techniques is not included in this text. The reader is referred to literature where they are well documented.

When the child begins to walk, exercises are begun to maintain the elongated position of the gastroc-soleus group and the evertors. Exercises to strengthen underdeveloped gastrocnemius and peronei muscles should be daily ritual. Shoes for clubfoot and lateral sole and heel wedges will improve the gait and maintain the corrected forefoot and heel position.

TARSAL COALITION

Rigid flatfoot is frequently caused by an anomalous fusion of two or more tarsal bones. This coalition prevents movement between the two tarsal bones involved causing a static foot deformity. The fusion may be osseous, cartilaginous, or fibrous. The most common coalitions exist between the talus and calcaneus and between the calcaneus and the navicular (Fig. 84).

Diagnosis

Tarsal coalition may be asymptomatic. It probably exists from birth but rarely gives symptoms until late adolescence or early adulthood when trauma such as prolonged standing, prolonged marching, or jumping may induce symptoms. The pain undoubtedly results from the stress sustained by the remaining functioning joints due to the unyielding coalition.

X-ray examination of the osseous bridge is requested when the clinical picture suggests coalition as a possible diagnosis. Cartilaginous or fibrous coalitions are not seen on the x-ray films but are assumed from clinical evaluation of a rigid painful foot that does not respond to conservative treatment.

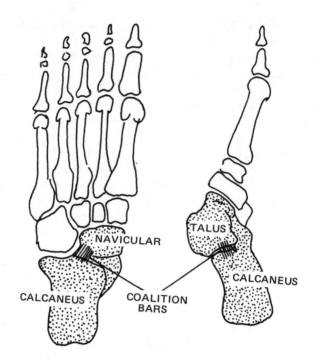

FIGURE 84. Tarsal coalition. Tarsal coalition is an anomalous fusion of two or more tarsal bones by a bony, cartilaginous, or fibrous bar. The most common types are talocalcaneal and calcaneonavicular. Their presence may form a rigid flatfoot or a peroneal "spastic" flatfoot. When the bar is bone it can be seen on x-ray film, otherwise its presence is diagnosed clinically.

Treatment

If trauma has produced mild discomfort, treatment is symptomatic and includes rest with heat applications. Immobilization of the foot and ankle in a walking plaster cast may be indicated to give complete rest and yet permit ambulation. If the coalition is considered to be the cause of the disability and persistent pain, resection of the bar or fusion stabilization of the subtalar joints may be necessary.

CALCANEOCAVUS FOOT

The cavus foot depends upon the apex of the deformity to be classified (Fig. 85). When the forefoot is cavus and all metatarsals are plantar flexed, the apex is at Chopart's joint and the condition is considered global. The local form of anterior cavus is when only the first metatarsal

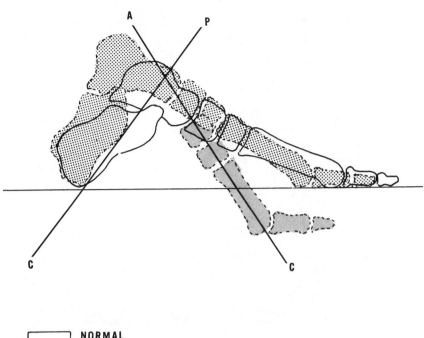

NORMAL

POSTERIOR CAVUS   P — C

ANTERIOR CAVUS   A — C

FIGURE 85. Types of calcaneocavus.

is vertical. The posterior calcaneocavus foot is the type in which the calcaneus is essentially vertical (in excess of 30°). Midfoot cavus is the type in which the apex is midtarsus posterior to the metatarsal cuneiform joint, but anterior to the tuberosity of the calcaneus. Any combination can exist.

Etiology

The usual cause of calcaneocavus foot is weakness of the gastroc-soleus (triceps sural) with strong ankle dorsiflexors (Fig. 86). This muscular imbalance occurs in conditions such as poliomyelitis, myelomeningocaele, or overcorrection of a heel cord lengthening. The ankle dorsiflexors acting through a long lever arm unopposed by the plantar flexors, rapidly cause a cavus condition. There is further shortening of the plantar fascia which accentuates the cavus.

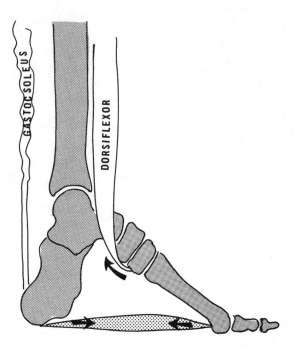

FIGURE 86. Muscles in calcaneocavus foot. Ragged lines indicate weakness of the gastroc-soleus; firm lines show strong ankle dorsiflexors.

Treatment

In the young child who is developing a calcaneocavus deformity, non-surgical treatment is usually ineffectual. Unless there is adequate strength of the gastroc-soleus, a nonoperative approach will be futile. No brace or orthotic device can prevent progressive deformity when there is a paralyzed gastroc-soleus.

Tendon transplant is a time-honored procedure but requires: (1) no fixed deformity, (2) transplanting a motor (muscle) that has adequate strength, and (3) no further return of function can be expected in the paretic plantar flexors of the foot and ankle. The transferred muscle must be functioning in as straight a line of pull as possible, and must be attached to bone. This requires no calcaneal varus or valgus. Tenodesis of the heel cord to the posterior fibula when there is no muscle suitable for transfer may create a slightly fixed equinus *which is far less disabling than a severe calcaneus.*

Tendon transplants must always consider whether the motor (muscle) has balanced varus or valgus effect. For example, transfer of peroneus longus to the calcaneus in the presence of a strong anterior tibialis will lead to inversion; thus, in addition to the peroneus transplant, the anterior tibialis should be moved to mid-foot to allow dorsiflexion but minimizing inversion of possible transfers. The peroneus brevis, peroneus longus, anterior tibialis, posterior tibial, flexor digitorum longus, or flexor hallucis longus all can be transferred to the calcaneus, but balance must be kept in mind and the ultimate strength of the transplanted muscles adequately replacing gastroc-soleus power.

The standard triple orthodesis should never be performed until the child is at least 10 years old to avoid excessive shortening of the foot. This orthodesis, however, is at best a salvage procedure.

When the foot has developed a fixed cavus deformity, osteotomy of the calcaneus has merit. There are numerous procedures but this text cannot detail all the procedures or evaluate their efficacy.

CONGENITAL VERTICAL TALUS

This uncommon condition should be suspected when the foot of the newborn is fixed in equinus and abduction. As the foot is dorsiflexed, the head of the talus forms a prominence at the expected longitudinal arch concavity similar to a rocker bottom foot and resembles a clubfoot improperly casted. X-ray films reveal the vertical talus.

Treatment

Treatment by manipulation and plaster casting is indicated but unfortunately is usually disappointing. The improvement is often merely in the appearance but not in the function of the foot. Surgical correction offers the most benefit.

BIBLIOGRAPHY

ADAMS, JC: *Outline of Orthopaedics*, ed 9. Churchill Livingston, New York, 1981.

CAILLIET, R: *Bracing for spasticity.* In LICHT, S (ED): *Orthotics Etcetera, Physical Medicine Library,* Vol 9. Elizabeth Licht, Publisher, New Haven, 1966, p 365.

DU VRIES, HL: *Surgery of the Foot*, ed 2. CV Mosby, St. Louis, 1965.

GARTLAND, JJ: *Fundamentals of Orthopaedics.* WB Saunders, Philadelphia, 1965.

GREEN, WT AND GRICE, DS: *The management of calcaneus deformity.* Am Acad Orthop Surg, Instructional Course Lectures, Vol 13: 135, 1956.

HARK, FW: *Rocker-foot due to congenital subluxation of the talus.* J Bone Joint Surg 32A: 344, 1950.

HENDERSON, WH AND CAMPBELL, JW: *The UC-BL Shoe Insert: Casting and Fabrication.* Biomechanics Laboratory of the University of California, July 1964.

HUTTER, CG AND SCOTT, W: *Tibial torsion.* J Bone Joint Surg 31-A: 511, 1949.

KITE, JH: *Congenital metatarsus varus. Report of 300 cases.* J Bone Joint Surg 32-A: 500, 1950.

KITE, JH: *Shoes for children.* In LICHT, S (ED): *Orthotics Etcetera. Physical Medicine Library, Vol 9.* Elizabeth Licht, Publisher, New Haven, 1966, p 453.

LEIBOLT, FL: *Shoes for children. Symposium in pediatric orthopedics.* Pediatr Clin North Am, 1955.

LEWIN, P: *The Foot and Ankle,* ed 4. Lea & Febiger, Philadelphia, 1959.

MACCONAILL, MA: *The postural mechanism of the human foot.* Proceedings of the Royal Irish Academy 1B:265, May 1945.

MCCAULEY, J, JR, LUSKIN, R, AND BROMLEY, J: *Recurrence in congenital metatarsus varus.* J Bone Joint Surg 46-A: 525, 1964.

NORTON, PL: *Pediatric orthopedics. Symposium in pediatric orthopedics.* Pediatr Clin North Am, 1955.

PONSETI, IV AND BECKER, JR: *Congenital metatarsus adductus. The results of treatment.* J Bone Joint Surg 48-A: 702, 1966.

SAMILSON, RL: *Calcaneocavus feet: A plan of management in children.* Orthopedic Review, Vol X, No 9: 121, 1951.

VAUGHN, WH AND SEGAL, G: *Tarsal coalition with special reference to roentgenographic interpretation.* Radiology 60:855, 1953.

WEBSTER, FS AND ROBERTS, WM: *Tarsal anomalies and peroneal spastic flatfoot.* JAMA 146: 1099, 1951.

WESTON, GW: *Tendon transfers about the foot, ankle and hip in the paralyzed lower extremity.* J Bone Joint Surg 47-A: 1430, 1965.

CHAPTER 6

Painful Disorders
of the Adult Foot

NORMAL FOOT

The *normal foot* conforms to the following criteria: (1) free of pain, (2) normal muscle balance, (3) absence of contracture, (4) three-point weight bearing, (5) a central heel, and (6) straight and mobile toes.

The majority of painful conditions of the foot originate in the soft tissues: the muscles, ligaments, tendons, nerves, and blood vessels. Articular and skeletal causes may be present from congenital abnormalities, infections, neoplasms, or trauma, but even in these cases the early symptoms come from soft-tissue changes.

In most cases of foot and ankle pain, the symptoms can be explained by local lesions. Usually, the area of pain pointed out by the patient specifies its exact anatomic site. The history gives the mechanism producing pain. Only rarely is foot pain referred from a proximal site, but the examiner must be aware that a local disturbance, such as flatfoot, may be an incidental finding in cases in which the pain is referred.

FOOT STRAIN

Foot strain may be acute, subacute, or chronic. It may occur in the normal foot from normal walking or standing if the patient has been unaccustomed to a great deal of activity. Since foot strain has a mechanical effect on the soft tissues, if it is allowed to persist, deformity may result. A foot considered mechanically abnormal may be strained by essentially normal activity. Stress on a pre-existing deformity will cause earlier and more intense pain and the foot will resist correction and palliation. The general rule that applies to all musculoskeletal dysfunctions applies here; that is, pain and dysfunction can occur from (1) abnormal stress on a normal structure, (2) normal stress on an abnormal structure,

105

or (3) normal stress on a normal structure when the structure is not prepared for the stress.

The static foot is supported by ligamentous tissues. There is no muscular activity in the foot or leg muscles during standing, even when large weights are superimposed upon the body. The muscular activity during locomotion prevents excessive strain upon the supportive ligaments and joint tissues. Therefore, pain in the static foot must result from faulty mechanics or an overwhelming stress upon the ligaments. In the moving foot, pain results when muscular incompetence due to disuse, imbalance, or abuse places an excessive burden upon the ligaments. In either case, the stress upon the soft tissues causes inflammation, elongation, and ultimately degeneration of the ligaments.

Acute Foot Strain

Acute painful ligamentous strain is usually self-limited, subsides with rest, and rarely presents a therapeutic problem. The acute situation is exemplified in the person paying an unaccustomed visit to a museum, the weekend athlete, or the doctor visiting the many booths at an annual convention. Rest followed by a gradual return to normal activities leads to recovery.

Chronic Foot Strain

If excessive stress is repeated or if normal stress is imposed upon a mechanical abnormality, the symptoms may become chronic. Symptoms may vary from those of ligamentous strain to those caused by joint malalignment resulting from the stress. Ultimately degenerative arthritic changes may be the source of pain.

The "breakdown" process follows a sequence. Ligaments exposed to chronic strain elongate and undergo inflammatory changes which result in pain. If the condition persists, the ligaments elongate and degenerate, lose their supporting function, and permit excessive motion of the joints. This excessive "play" and misalignment of the joints will inflame the joint capsules and surfaces, and articular inflammation becomes the source of pain. If irritation to the joints continues, structural damage to the articular surfaces results, and degenerative arthritis is present. Nature responds to these irritations by attempting reconstruction or forming a bulwark against the irritation with an overgrowth of bone that results in a deformed joint called an "arthrosis." If early changes are recognized, this cycle is reversible, but if it is allowed to proceed too far, the joint may be beyond repair.

The initial symptom of acute stress from activity such as prolonged walking is muscular fatigue, usually described as an "aching" in the sole

106

of the foot, calf muscles, or occasionally the anterior leg. Deep tenderness of the plantar tissues of the foot or the leg muscles is found. The foot, now symptomatic, may be normal but is more likely to be a pronated foot which flattens its longitudinal arch upon weight bearing. Muscular fatigue from activity permits stress to be imposed upon the ligaments resulting in ligamentous pain (Fig. 87).

Mechanism and Sequence

The mechanism and sequence by which strain is imposed upon the areas of the foot are illustrated in Figures 88 and 89. The foot and ankle must be considered as a complex structure with each of its component parts dependent upon the others. Body weight is borne upon the talus through its articulation with the tibia. In turn, the talus is supported by the calcaneus and is held in an oblique manner. The oblique seating of the talus upon the calcaneus gives the talus a tendency to *glide forward* and *medially upon the calcaneus.* The resultant force of this movement forces the calcaneus into eversion and depresses its anterior portion. This prona-

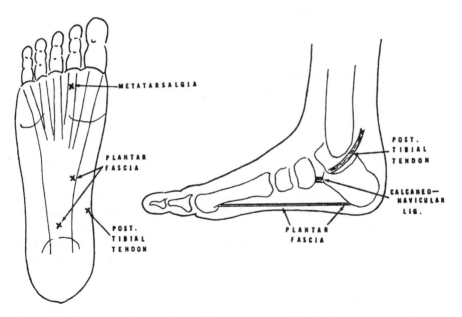

FIGURE 87. Tender areas in foot strain. "Trigger areas" noted in the foot undergoing strain. The initial tenderness is usually noted on the medial border of the plantar fascia and later near the heel. The deltoid ligament is not shown, but is a point of tenderness near the posterior tibial tendon which becomes strained. The second metatarsal head is the most prevalent site of metatarsalgia.

107

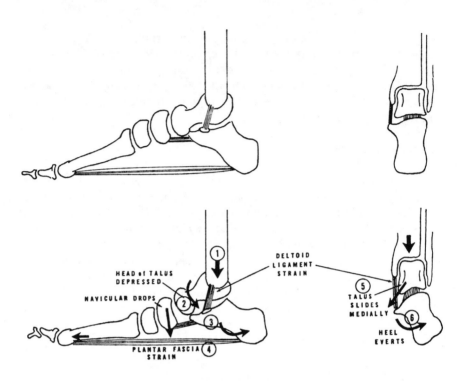

FIGURE 88. Mechanism and sequence of foot strain. The upper figures depict the normal foot with proper bone and joint alignment, adequate longitudinal arch, and a central heel. *(1)* The weight-bearing stress imparted through the tibia upon the talus *(2)* which slides forward and medially *(5)* upon the supporting calcaneus. The calcaneus *(3)* is depressed anteriorly elongating the entire foot, thus placing strain upon the plantar ligaments *(4)*. The calcaneus everts under the downward pressure of the talus and goes into valgus *(6)*.

tion depresses the longitudinal arch and stretches the plantar ligament and fascia.

The valgus position of the heel places a torque stress upon the forefoot, which responds by becoming everted. The foot now bears the weight on its inner border, which forces the foot into more pronation thus placing strain on the medial ankle ligaments and upon the tendon of the posterior tibial muscle. Due to the valgus heel position, the Achilles tendon deviates laterally and shortens. The shortened tendon places more strain upon the anterior segments of the foot.

Pronation

This sequence of effects of foot strain may be imposed upon a normal foot but is more apt to occur in the already pronated or deconditioned

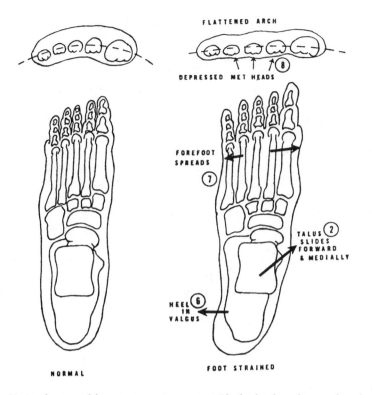

FLATTENED ARCH

DEPRESSED MET HEADS

FOREFOOT
SPREADS

TALUS
SLIDES
FORWARD
& MEDIALLY

HEEL
IN
VALGUS

NORMAL

FOOT STRAINED

FIGURE 89. Mechanism of foot strain: superior view. The heel is forced into valgus from the downward pressure of the superincumbant talus *(2)*. This causes the forefoot to abduct (evert) and spread out *(7)*. The normal transverse arch flattens and depresses the central metatarsal heads *(8)*.

foot. As the protective muscular action is overwhelmed, the stress is imparted upon the ligaments, then the joint capsules, and ultimately the joints. Joints so strained separate slightly, and the foot undergoes a functional deformity. Persistence of the stress ultimately converts the functional deformity into a structural one. Recovery from an acute strain is brief if the tissues are healthy and mobile. If the strain is chronic or the tissues are defective, deformity becomes chronic and subsequent stresses although minor can elicit major symptoms.

During the early phase of strain upon the foot, the muscles acting across the foot attempt to allay the strain upon the ligaments. They may react to this stress with pain. The posterior tibial tendon, as the prime invertor of the foot, opposes the eversion of the foot, and its tendon may become inflamed and tender. On examination, tenderness of the posterior tibial tendon can be elicited by palpation along its course under and behind the medial malleolus (see Fig. 87). The long flexor of the big toe,

109

which has a function similar to the posterior tibial and also presses the toe to the ground, also becomes strained and painfully inflamed.

As the foot and forefoot go more into pronation, the lateral evertors must shorten to take up the slack. The peronei muscles and toe extensors, the evertors, go into "spasm" as they undergo adaptive shortening, and they too become painful and tender.

The interosseous talocalcaneal ligament which binds the talus to the calcaneus (see Fig. 8) is normally taut when the foot is supinated and slack when the foot is pronated. As the strained foot pronates, the tarsal canal deforms and the talocalcaneal joint becomes abnormally mobile. Although slack, the interosseous ligament undergoes strain with ultimate inflammation. This tender ligament can be palpated at the lateral orifice of the sinus canal just anterior to the lateral malleolus (see Fig. 40). Tenderness of this ligament occurs late in the sequence as the foot undergoes pronation deformity.

Early ligamentous symptoms are felt on the plantar surface of the foot (see Fig. 87) with the areas of tenderness palpable in the plantar fascia, the medial ligaments of the ankle at their attachment to the sustentaculum talus (see Figs. 6 and 39), and the posterior tibial tendon passing under the medial malleolus.

Diagnosis

The early signs and symptoms in the soft tissues that relate to structural surface anatomy (see Figs. 38 to 40) are pointed to by the patient and ascertained by the examiner. Functional anatomy gives a mechanical explanation by which abnormal function results in pain and disability. It is evident that pronation is a major cause of pain, and that deconditioning as well as excessive stress initiates a process of decompensation. This emphasizes the need for a long-range program of treatment for children with markedly pronated feet to allay ultimate pain and disability in adulthood.

The toe flexors, as well as the supinators of the foot, play a vital role in the maintenance of the longitudinal and transverse arches. Balance between the toe flexors and extensors must exist for proper foot function. Normally, the extensor digitorum longus and the lumbricals extend the distal interphalangeal joints (Fig. 90) and the toe flexors press the straightened toes against the floor. This action elevates the transverse arch. If the intrinsics are weak, the phalanges are permitted to flex, and the action of the toe flexors causes a "claw" position of the toes. The metatarsal heads become more prominent and weight-bearing. With weakness of the toe flexors, the downward pressure upon the floor is also weakened.

The excessive joint "play" resulting from ligamentous laxity causes pain due to articular strain. The calcaneocuboid and the talonavicular joints

110

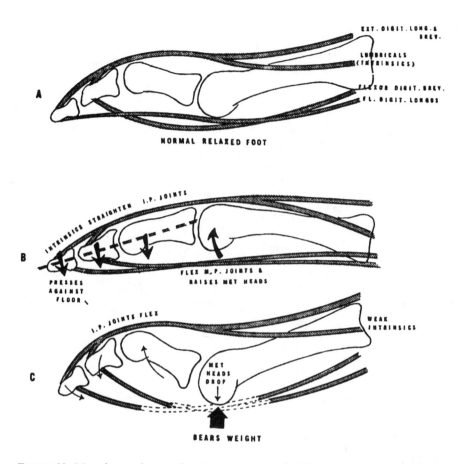

FIGURE 90. Muscular mechanism forming transverse arch. The transverse arch is only a potential arch, not an anatomic arch. The metatarsal heads are raised by the toes being kept straight and the metatarsophalangeal joints being flexed *(B)* by the long and short flexors. Weakness of the intrinsics permits the toes to bend at the interphalangeal joints, and the flexors then increase the flexion at the interphalangeal joints. The metatarsal heads thus bear the full-body weight.

(Fig. 91) sustain this stress primarily by virtue of the foot pronating and the forefoot everting.

Pain originating from articular strain does not subside with rest as does pain from ligamentous, tendinous, or muscular origin. No "trigger" areas are palpable, and the patient points to a region overlying the joint involved. Pain can be reproduced by forcefully everting the forefoot while immobilizing the heel.

Talonavicular arthrosis resulting from chronic foot strain causes tenderness over the dorsum of the foot at the talonavicular joint, and because

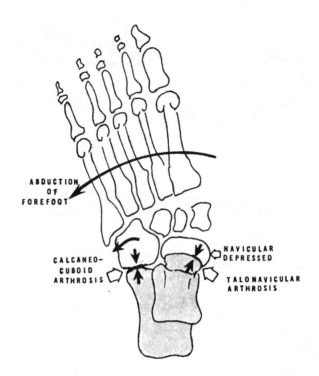

FIGURE 91. The chronically strained foot. The abducted forefoot of the chronically strained foot causes articular changes due to pressure of the abducted cuboid upon the calcaneus. The talus drops and causes pressure upon the superior portion of the navicular. Mechanical pressures at joints cause arthrosis.

the navicular is depressed in the pronated foot, there is also tenderness on the plantar surface of the foot at the calcaneonavicular ligament.

Treatment

Treatment of foot strain is essentially the treatment of the adult flatfoot. In acute strain, rest is desirable and walking must be curtailed or completely eliminated. Application of heat or cold may be used depending upon which affords the greater relief. Early use of cold, and later the use of heat is generally preferred. The use of alternating hot and cold baths is soothing. Stimulation of the plantar muscles with faradic current allegedly affords comfort by decreasing the soft-tissue inflammation. When the symptoms are sufficiently severe or fail to respond to brief rest, immobilization of the foot in a plaster cast may be indicated. A cast removes all stress from the intrinsic muscles of the foot and gives total rest while still permitting ambulation.

112

After the acute symptoms have subsided, rehabilitation of the foot must be undertaken. Often the patient's history indicates that pain began after a change in occupation, a change in activities involving excessive standing or walking, a period of excessive weight gain, or a period of immobilization causing disuse wasting of the muscles. It is not unusual to find that symptoms began with the wearing of a different type of shoe. These factors are very often the cause of foot pain and once discovered must be altered or remedied.

Exercises similar to those given the child with pronated feet (Chapter 5) are extremely valuable for patients up to the age of 50 and can be of value even at a later stage in life. These exercises preferably are done barefooted. While seated, the patient turns the foot down, in, up, and out drawing a wide circle. This must be done forcefully, with every effort to get the fullest possible range of motion. Simultaneously, the toes should be alternately flexed and extended. This type of exercise elongates the tissues and strengthens the muscles of the leg and foot. Circulation is also enhanced.

Similar exercises can be performed standing. The patient stands with feet apart and slight toeing in. Rolling to the outer border of the feet, the patient simultaneously curls the toes forcefully. Rising on the toes strengthens the calf group and the toe flexors, and the patient should be encouraged to practice walking on his toes with a slight pigeon-toed gait. If the heel cord is tight, it can be stretched by the exercise shown in Figure 41 in which the patient leans forward against a wall, keeping one leg behind, and the forward leg not weight-bearing. The posterior foot is kept facing straight ahead with the heel to the ground. As the patient leans toward the wall, the Achilles tendon is stretched. The toe flexors can be exercised by wrinkling a towel lying on the floor or picking up marbles with the toes.

All the exercises prescribed are of value when done daily and systematically for long periods. The patient should do these exercises while wearing shoes during the work day. The patient must be advised to walk with a slight toe-in gait and with a slight spring during push-off. Most *important of all, the patient must walk increasing distances daily.*

Corrective shoes in the adult seek to decrease the strain causing pronation. An adult foot in which the abnormal articular structure is fixed cannot be modified, as can a child's or an adult's whose foot is flexible. The shoe is modified by elevating the inner border using a Thomas heel with an inner wedge of $1/8$ to $3/16$ inch. An inner wedge may also be incorporated into the sole to raise the entire inner border of the shoe.

Tape with $1/4$ inch adhesive-backed sponge rubber can be applied to elevate the portion of the foot desired. Several layers of moleskin or felt of varying thicknesses cut into the desired pattern and taped properly to the foot is also effective (Fig. 92).

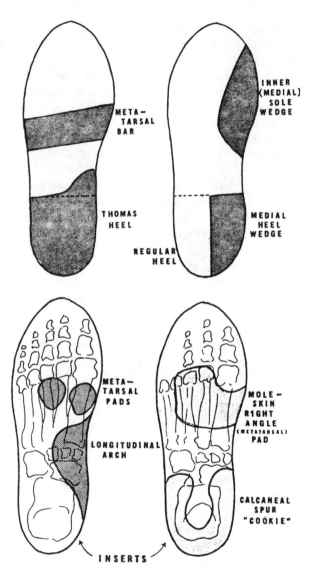

FIGURE 92. Shoe modifications to correct strain factors.

Arch supports may help rehabilitate the flexible flatfoot. They must be molded to conform to the shape of the foot that is partially weight-bearing, yet properly formed; they are never molded to the shape of the non-weight-bearing foot. They must be sufficiently firm to support the body weight without completely deforming. The shoe must be large enough to accommodate both the arch supports and the foot.

Shoes must be fitted properly. As foot tone is best in the morning and the foot "spreads" and slightly deforms as the day progresses, shoes should be fitted late in the day. The shoe should be broad across the forefoot, have a firm-fitting counter, and have a last that conforms to the weight-bearing print of the foot. It should be long enough to project 1 inch ahead of the big toe. Women's shoes should have broad low heels, rounded toes, and a vamp that will not constrict the metatarsal heads. It is a sad commentary that women's shoes are designed exclusively for style and custom, with no concern for comfort and health.

METATARSALGIA

Metatarsalgia is a symptom of pain in the forefoot. It is essentially pain and tenderness of the plantar heads of the metatarsal bones that bear a disproportionate amount of the body weight.

In normal gait, at "heel strike," the moment of ground contact that ends the swing phase and begins the stance phase, the foot is inverted due to anterior tibial muscle function. As the foot progresses through the stance phase, the weight bearing progresses along the outer aspect of the foot and gradually across the metatarsal heads until the last phase of stance, when the foot pronates due to the weight-bearing torque of tibial internal torsion (see Chapter 3). In static stance, the first metatarsal carries two sixths of the body weight (Fig. 93) and the others one sixth each. In a pronated or "splayed" foot, the balance is upset. The transverse arch depresses and greater weight is borne on the second, third, and fourth metatarsal heads (Fig. 94). The interosseous ligaments that support the arch are stretched, permitting the forefoot to broaden and "splay" out.

Metatarsalgia is not an anatomic diagnosis, and may be divided into primary and secondary metatarsalgia. *Primary metatarsalgia* may be (1) static, (2) congenital, (3) long first ray, (4) secondary to hallux valgus, or (5) secondary to surgery of the foot for other conditions. *Secondary metatarsalgia* may result from (1) trauma, (2) sesamoiditis, or (3) neurogenic disorders.

Diagnosis

At first there is tenderness over the metatarsal heads. This may be described by the patient as "walking with a pebble in the shoe." Ultimately, a callus forms over the second or third metatarsal head, which is itself painful, and aggravates the irritation by increasing the weight bearing upon the metatarsal head. The tenderness is noted by the examiner squeezing the metatarsal head between the thumb and index finger. The

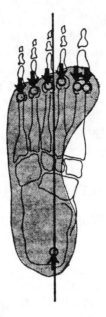

FIGURE 93. Static foot: weight-bearing points. There are six weight-bearing points of the metatarsal heads. Due to the two sesamoid bones, the first metatarsal carries two-sixths of the weight. This balance is upset in the pronated or splay foot.

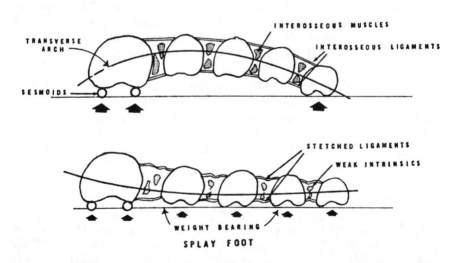

FIGURE 94. Splay foot. A constitutional weakness of the intermetatarsal ligament combined with weakness of the intrinsic muscles of the foot may cause the foot to spread excessively under weight bearing. Symptoms consist of pressure pain of the middle metatarsal heads with formation of bunions and calluses.

examiner must compress each metatarsal head individually and must *not* compress the tissues between the heads. This space contains ligaments and the interdigital nerves and can confuse the examiner.

Metatarsalgia is common in the middle aged who have a pronation tendency and most common after a weight gain. This combination and increasing sedentary existence, increases symptomatology. Internal tibial torsion or knock-knees can increase the pronation of the foot. A "toe-out" gait increases pronation.

The pronated foot is a loose packed articular forefoot in that all the joints are incongruous and the articulations widened to permit the foot to splay (spread). This also permits the transverse metatarsal head arch to float. This causes a wider print of the wet foot upon absorbing paper, as the arch depresses in the same manner as flatfoot.

As the foot everts, from whatever causes the anterior tibialis muscle that inverts (supinates), the foot is less efficient. The toe extensors now are in direct alignment of the foot and function more to dorsiflex the foot. This further everts the foot, and simultaneously dorsiflexes (extends) the proximal phalanges. The extended proximal phalanx further exposes the metatarsal heads to excessive depression and weight bearing.

Treatment

Metatarsalgia, caused by a depressed transverse arch is treated by elevating the middle portion of the arch, which avoids pressure on the painful metatarsal heads. All the aspects of treating the pronated foot must be utilized including exercises to strengthen the intrinsic muscles, Achilles tendon stretching, improvement of gait, weight reduction, and the use of appliances such as the Thomas heel, the inner heel wedge, and the metatarsal pad (see Fig. 92). The metatarsal pad must be placed *behind* the metatarsal heads to relieve the pressure on them. If it is placed *under* the heads, a frequent error made by the orthotist or shoe repairman, the condition will be aggravated (Fig. 95). Calluses must be treated by soaking the foot in warm water and then using a stone or emery board. However, to administer all these ancillary forms of treatment and not correct the abnormal mechanics of the foot is to invite recurrence.

SPLAY FOOT

Splay foot is essentially a broadened forefoot due to weakness of the intermetatarsal ligaments associated with weakness of the intrinsic muscles (see Fig. 94). The transverse arch flattens and the middle metatarsal heads bear more than the usual amount of weight. Calluses form on the plantar surfaces of the heads. Hammer toes may form because of the excessive extension of the toes and cause pain and tenderness on the dor-

117

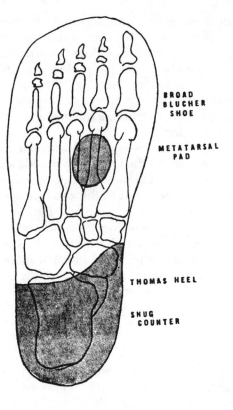

FIGURE 95. Shoe modifications in treatment of metatarsalgia. Placement of the metatarsal pad to elevate the heads of the second and third metatarsals must be *behind* the metatarsal heads. The broad forefoot shoe and a soft upper permits spreading of the foot without cramping, and the soft upper prevents calluses from forming on the dorsum of the toes. If a Thomas heel is used, the counter must be snug to hold the heel centrally.

sum of the toe joints. Calluses may form here. The splay foot is not a specific entity but usually accompanies the pronated foot. It more aptly applies to a broad flexible forefoot and a minor degree of pronation. Treatment is the same as for the pronated foot.

FREIBERG'S DISEASE

Ischemic epiphyseal necrosis of the second metatarsal was initially described by Freiberg and Kohler. This disease occurs in adolescents before they have complete epiphyseal closure of the metatarsals. It is similar to Legg-Calvé-Perthes disease (ischemic necrosis of the epiphysis of the femoral head) and, as in that disease, there is no specific known cause except

118

avascular necrosis of an unclosed epiphysis. Freiberg's disease occurs in adolescence but may be asymptomatic until adulthood when there is deformity of the involved toe and degenerative arthritis of that metacarpophalangeal joint. It usually involves the second metatarsal but may occur at the third.

Diagnosis

Diagnosis is confirmed by x-ray films showing characteristic changes suggested by pain and tenderness of the second metatarsal head. The metaphyseal changes occur in the dorsal position of the metaphysis and the changes result in the head moving dorsally (Fig. 96).

Treatment

Treatment consists of prolonged conservative management using an orthotic metatarsal platform, exercises, and contrast baths. Later, if con-

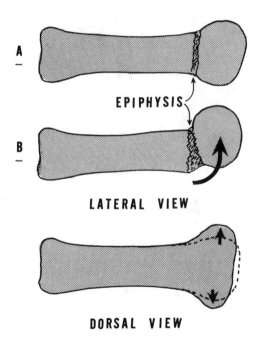

FIGURE 96. Freiberg's disease (crushing osteochondrosis). *A* depicts the normal metatarsal bone in the adolescent with its emphyseal growth plate. In *B*, there has been an epiphysitis and the upward pressure causes the head to migrate dorsally. It fuses in this position and the head (dorsal view) widens. Pain and disability may result. Condition occurs in the second metatarsal head.

servative measures fail to relieve symptoms and afford comfort, osteotomy or metatarsal head resection may be necessary.

SHORT FIRST TOE: MORTON'S SYNDROME

A short first metatarsal, termed Morton's syndrome (Dudley Morton), causes excessive weight to be borne by the second metatarsal head and is usually hereditary. Morton's syndrome consists of (1) an excessively short first metatarsal, which is hypermobile at its base where it articulates with the second metatarsal and the cuneiform, (2) posterior displacement of the sesamoids, and (3) thickening of the second metatarsal shaft (Fig. 97).

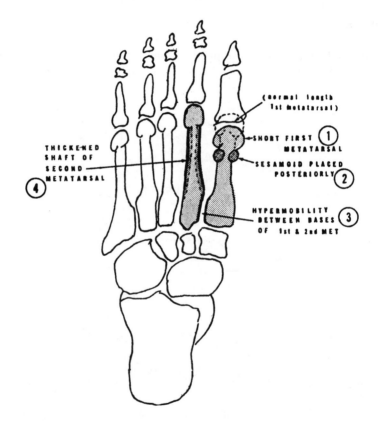

FIGURE 97. The short first metatarsal: Dudley Morton syndrome. This syndrome of metatarsalgia consists of *(1)* a shorter than normal first metatarsal, *(2)* posterior displacement of the sesamoid bones, *(3)* excessive mobility of the first metatarsal at its base, and *(4)* thickening of the shaft of the second metatarsal as a result of excessive weight bearing imposed upon this bone. The pain and tenderness is usually felt at the *base* of the first two metatarsals and the *head* of the second.

120

Diagnosis

The additional weight borne by the second metatarsal causes excessive mobility at its base and strain of the ligaments, capsules, and muscles where the metatarsal articulates with the cuneiform and the second metatarsal. Calluses form under the second and third metatarsals because the transverse arch is also depressed.

Treatment

Treatment consists of building a "platform" under the first metatarsal bone to assume the weight and relieve the second metatarsal. The other forms of treating pronated foot are also indicated for Morton's syndrome.

Morton's syndrome (Dudley Morton) should not be confused with Morton's metatarsalgia (Thomas G. Morton). Morton's metatarsalgia is basically a neuralgia due to an interdigital neoplasm. This is a fibrous thickening of the digital nerve usually between the third and fourth metatarsals and is fully discussed in Chapter 11 (Fig. 122).

MARCH FRACTURE

Diagnosis

March fracture is a stress fracture of a metatarsal bone. Pain, often noted after a long march, is the presenting symptom. A history of violent injury is rare, making the cause difficult to pinpoint. The pathology is a hairline fracture of the shaft of the second or third metatarsal with no displacement of the fragments. Initially, the fracture may not be revealed by routine x-ray examination, but later callous formation around the fracture is radiologically apparent (Fig. 98) and confirms the diagnosis.

Clinically, there is tenderness at the middle of the shaft involved and pain is evoked by flexion or extension of the toes. Pain subsides with rest and non-weight bearing and recurs with exertion. Repeated weight bearing causes swelling and redness at the fracture site. When the history fails to elicit trauma and x-ray examination fails to reveal a fracture, the first view of the callus on the x-ray film raises the suspicion of a sarcoma.

Treatment

Treatment of the march fracture is symptomatic as this type of fracture heals spontaneously. If pain is severe, a walking plaster cast applied for four weeks will give relief.

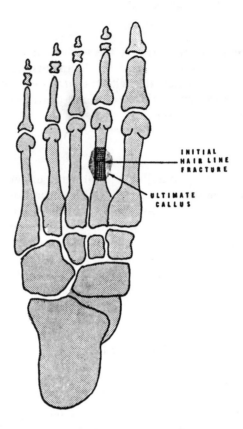

INITIAL
HAIR LINE
FRACTURE

ULTIMATE
CALLUS

FIGURE 98. March fracture of the second metatarsal. The initial fracture is often not observed in routine x-ray examination or appears as a thin hair-line fracture. Within three weeks, after persistent pain, swelling, and tenderness, the callous formation indicative of healing becomes evident radiologically. This may be the first positive diagnostic sign. Displacement of fragments is rare.

PES CAVUS

Pes cavus, also termed clawfoot, pes arcuatus, or hollow foot (Fig. 99), is a foot with an unusually high arch. The high longitudinal arch causes shortening of the foot, and the obliquity of the metatarsals to the floor causes increased pressure on the metatarsal heads with resultant calluses. Due to the high convex arch, the extensor ligaments are relatively shortened causing dorsiflexion of the proximal phalanges. The distal phalanges are plantar flexed resulting in clawing of the toes. Calluses form on the dorsum of the toes as well as under the heads. The metatarsophalangeal joints frequently dislocate and the forefoot is usually inflexible.

122

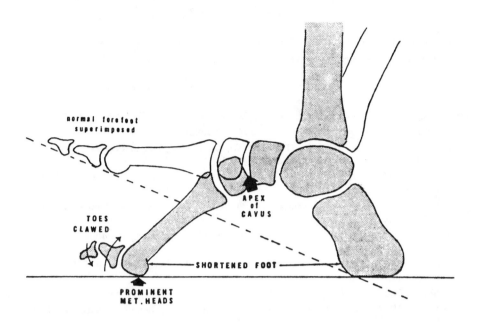

FIGURE 99. Pes cavus. The pes cavus foot has an exaggerated longitudinal arch with its apex at the naviculocuneiform joint. The foot is shorter than normal, the metatarsal heads are prominent, and the toes clawed. The clawing of the toes is due to contracture of the toe extensors. The distal phalanges are flexed and there are dislocations of the metatarso-phalangeal joints. Slanting the illustration until the floor (dotted line) is horizontal depicts the superimposed normal foot.

A very high cavus foot may be totally asymptomatic and symptoms, when they exist, are those of pressure upon the metatarsal heads or unusual fatigue when walking or standing. Mildly symptomatic pes cavus is treated with properly fitted shoes with a low heel and a metatarsal bar (see Fig. 92). Exercises to stretch the toe extensors and distal toe flexors are recommended. Surgery of soft tissues, such as a plantar fasciotomy or tendon transplant, is usually unsuccessful. Osteotomies to reshape the foot may be required in severe symptomatic cases.

SUMMARY

There are obviously many other causes of foot pain in the adult that cannot be given full discussion in this text. They include fractures, dislocations, neoplastic growths, and infections. Each would require specific consideration that is relegated to the numerous texts available to the interested physician.

BIBLIOGRAPHY

ADAMS, JC: *Outline of Orthopaedics*, ed 9. Churchill Livingston, New York, 1981.

BAILEY, H: *Demonstrations of Physical Signs in Clinical Surgery*, ed 13. Williams & Wilkins, Baltimore, 1960.

BARNETT, CH, DAVIES, DV, AND MACCONAILL, MA: *Synovial Joints: Their Structure and Mechanics*. Charles C Thomas, Springfield, Ill, 1961.

BASMAJIAN, JV: *Man's Posture*. Archives of Physical Medicine 46:26, 1965.

DUVRIES, HL: *Surgery of the Foot*. CV Mosby, St Louis, 1965.

FREEMAN, MA, DEAN, MR, AND HANHAM, IW: *The etiology and prevention of functional instability of the foot*. J Bone Joint Surg 47:678, 1965.

FREIBERG, AH: *Interaction of the second metatarsal bone*. Surg Gynecol Obstet 19:191, 1914.

FREIBERG, AH: *The so-called infarction of the second metatarsal bone*. J Bone Joint Surg 8:257, 1926.

KAPLAN, E: *Some principles of anatomy and kinesiology in stabilizing operations of the foot*. Clin Orthop 34:7, 1964.

KOHLER, A: *Typical disease of the second metatarsophalangeal joint*. Am J Roentgenol 10:705, 1923.

LICHT, S: *Therapeutic Exercises*. Elizabeth Licht, Publisher, New Haven, 1958.

MILGRAM, JE: *Office measures for relief of the painful foot*. J Bone Joint Surg 46-A:1096, 1964.

RUBIN, G AND WITTEN, M: *The talar-tilt angle and the fibular collateral ligaments: A method for the determination of talar tilt*. J Bone Joint Surg 42-A:311, 1960.

WILSON, JN: *The treatment of deformities of the foot and toes*. Br J Phys Med 17:4, 1954.

ZAMOSKY, I: *Shoe modifications in lower-extremity orthotics*. Bull Prosthet Res 10:2, Fall 1964.

ZAMOSKY, I AND LICHT, S: *Shoes and their modifications*. In LICHT, S (ED): *Orthotics Etcetera, Physical Medicine Library*, Vol 9. Elizabeth Licht, Publisher, New Haven, 1966, p 388.

CHAPTER 7

The Foot in Rheumatoid Arthritis

RHEUMATOID ARTHRITIS

The systemic manifestations of rheumatoid arthritis, particularly the hand and upper extremity involvement, are stressed but the foot in rheumatoid arthritis does not get proportionate consideration. Foot involvement in rheumatoid arthritis is both painful and disabling.

The etiology and diagnosis of rheumatoid arthritis will not be stressed here, as there is already a great deal of written information on the subject. This text concerns itself only with foot and ankle involvement.

Synovitis

The mechanism of synovitis, its involvement of articular tissues, and its relationship to joints in the foot are discussed here. The initial pathology is currently considered to be an antigen-antibody immune reaction, with invasion of polymorphonuclear (PMN) leucocytes at the tissue site to be the pathology. These PMN leucocytes attack the cartilage and release lysosomal enzymes that cause synovitis and degeneration of the cartilage. The synovial inflammatory reaction results in granular tissue formation, which furthers cartilage erosion. The lysosomal absorption of cartilage and the invasion of the cartilage by granular tissue is the basis of rheumatoid arthritic pathology of joints.

Cartilage varies as to its site of invasion and damage and, therefore, differs as to the type of joint involved (Fig. 100). Where a joint has contact with opposing cartilage, the apex of cartilage at the site of contact undergoes the least damage. Peripherally, where the synovium contacts the cartilage there is greater damage to the cartilage, and where the synovium reflects upon itself, there is the greatest degree of damage.

The greatest degree of inflammation with formation of villus occurs at the peripheral folds. Early x-ray studies of rheumatoid arthritis reveal

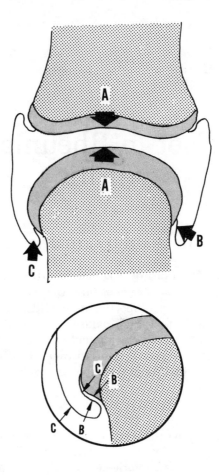

FIGURE 100. Rheumatoid arthritis: joint site involvement. *(A)*, Least damage occurs at site of direct compression. *(B)*, Fold of synovium upon cartilage is the site of greater damage. *(C)*, Fold of synovium upon cartilage is the site of greatest damage.

erosion of the joints at these sites. The invading villus is florid and can completely undermine the cartilage. The overlying pannus can completely cover and erode the cartilage surface (Fig. 101).

The joint capsule and its supporting ligament also become invaded by inflammatory synovium and stretch, allowing the joint to sublux or dislocate. In the foot, the tendons of peronei, tibialis anterior, tibialis posterior, and the toe extensors can be invaded and ultimately rupture. If there is sufficient synovial swelling in the tarsal tunnel, nerve compression within the tunnel may cause nerve ischemia with a resultant neuropathy. This condition is described in Chapter 9, Painful Conditions of the Heel.

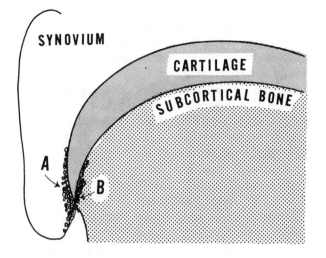

FIGURE 101. Villus formation in rheumatoid arthritis. *(A)*, Villus (pannus) covers the peripheral cartilage and digests it. *(B)*, Villus undermines the cartilage invading between it and the subcortical bone.

The collagen layering the muscle fibers may undergo inflammatory degeneration leading to atrophy, contraction, and fibrosis. This contracture of periarticular muscles combined with intra-articular capsular fibrosis can lead to a stiff joint.

The intrinsic muscles may undergo swelling during the acute stage forcing the toes to spread. When the muscles fibrose and contract they may cause clawing, that is, hyperextension of the proximal phalanx with compensatory flexion of the distal phalanx. The original spreading, followed by clawing, exposes the metatarsal head to weight-bearing pressure with resultant metatarsalgia. The transverse metatarsal arch may flatten or reverse, thus exposing the second, third, and fourth metatarsal heads to excessive weight bearing and pain. (See section on metatarsalgia in Chapter 6, Painful Disorders of the Adult Foot.)

In rheumatoid arthritis, even if untreated with steroids, osteoporosis is usual. These osteoporotic bones lead to mechanical complication. Rheumatoid vasculitis may occur leading to cutaneous or subcutaneous ischemia and skin breakdown. Rheumatoid neuropathy may also occur causing sensory loss with resultant trophic ulcers. The examiner of a rheumatoid arthritic patient, besides checking for occular and renal changes, must periodically *examine the feet for vascular, osseous, and peripheral nerve function as well as articular changes.*

CLINICAL RHEUMATOID ARTHRITIS

Changes in the metatarsal phalangeal joints with metatarsalgia is a frequent early rheumatologic sign. The mechanisms causing this condition are numerous. The intrinsic muscles swell when synovitis causes the forefoot to spread and contract when fibrosis causes "clawing" of the toes. The foot pronates as a result of attrition of the anterior tibialis. The toe extensors assume the dorsiflexion role with simultaneous eversion and further pronation and exposure of the metatarsal heads. Rheumatoid changes may also involve the knee, causing a valgus and further pronation of the foot. Early recognition of an incipient pronated foot and the metatarsalgia tendency must rely on full mechanical lower extremity evaluation and the institution of corrective measures. These have been innumerated in the pronated foot section in Chapter 6.

Interestingly, the ankle joint is involved to a lesser degree than is the foot, and disabling severity is not as great. There is much less synovium in the ankle joint and therefore less synovitis. Changes in the tarsal joints may cause less flexibility and thus impose more strain upon the talar-mortise articulartion. The talar joints must always be carefully and specifically evaluated as to mobility or involvement as well as determining the ankle range of motion.

Pain and limitation may occur in the tarsal joints causing a painful rigid pronated planus foot or a cavus foot. Clinical examination of mobility of each joint coupled with x-ray verification leads to recognition of these changes.

The foot of a rheumatoid arthritic patient must be evaluated in its relationship to the entire lower extremity as each component—the hip, the knee, the hindfoot, and the forefoot—influences the others.

When the hip exhibits a flexion contracture, the knee compensates with flexion and the ankle simultaneously compensates with ankle dorsiflexion. The gait, as well as the individual joints, must be evaluated. When the hip is internally or externally rotated, the knee ultimately assumes varus or valgus to compensate. The ankle and foot also assume compensatory postures or movements that may be detrimental. The foot abnormality of pronation or supination may be primary and may secondarily affect the knee and hip. Whichever joint is involved, treatment must be instituted early and energetically. *Total evaluation of the lower extremity and orthotic or surgical correction of all factors are necessary.*

BIBLIOGRAPHY

Currey, HLF: *Aetiology and pathogenesis of rheumatoid arthritis.* In Scott, JT (ed): *Capeman's Textbook of the Rheumatic Diseases,* ed 5. Churchill Livingston, New York, 1978.

FOWLER, AW: *A method of forefoot reconstruction*. J Bone Joint Surg 41B:507, 1959.

HELFET, AJ AND LEE, DMG: *Disorders of the Foot*. JB Lippincott, Philadelphia, 1980, p 159.

RAPES, MW, ET AL: *Diagnostic criteria for rheumatoid arthritis*. Ann Rheum Dis 18:49, 1959.

CHAPTER 8

Painful Abnormalities of the Toes

HALLUX VALGUS

Hallux valgus is the most common painful deformity of the big toe. Pathologically, it is a lateral deviation of the proximal phalanx on the first metatarsal. This condition is generally attributed to the forcing of a foot with a short first metatarsal, into a shoe with a pointed toe and high heel. In common usage, the symptomatic hallux valgus is termed "bunion," and the terms are used interchangeably.

Diagnosis

There are three components to the "bunion complex:" (1) the large toe angulates toward the second toe, (2) the medial portion of the first metatarsal head enlarges, and (3) the bursa over the medial aspect of the joint becomes inflamed and thick-walled (Fig. 102). This condition is found most frequently in older women who have a broadened forefoot, with a flattened transverse arch in a pronated foot. The big toe frequently overlies the second toe (Fig. 103).

Etiologic Concepts

There are many concepts regarding the etiology of hallux valgus. Congenital factors may exist that predispose to deformity in later life. The first metatarsal may be shorter and may be in varus as a residual of metatarsus primus varus (see Fig. 82) in childhood. The varus of the first metatarsal may be due to obliquity of the first cuneiform bone, which changes the angle of the first tarsometatarsal joint (Fig. 104A). The head of the first metatarsal may be more convex than normal and permit the first phalanx to shift laterally (see Fig. 104A). Primary or secondary mus-

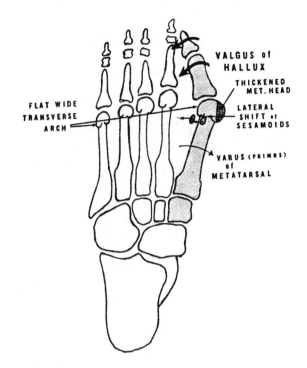

FIGURE 102. Hallux valgus. Hallux valgus is essentially a subluxation of the two phalanges of the big toe in a valgus direction. The first metatarsal deviates in a varus direction and the sesamoids are thus shifted laterally. These major bony and articular changes characterize hallux valgus.

cular imbalance will pull the first phalanx laterally and overcome the ineffectual abductor hallucis (Fig. 104C).

When the foot is forced into a high-heeled shoe with a pointed toe and permitted to pronate more from added body weight and debilitation of the intrinsic muscles, the first toe deviates increasingly in a lateral direction. The long tendons of the big toe, both flexor and extensor, shift laterally, along with the sesamoid bones and exert traction upon the big toe causing further valgus (Fig. 104B). There are many additional factors contributing to hallux valgus either as primary or secondary influences.

Treatment

Treatment of hallux valgus must be individualized and will depend on the age of the patient, the degree of deformity, and the severity and duration of the symptoms attributed to the hallux valgus. Many patients with severe deformity are free of symptoms.

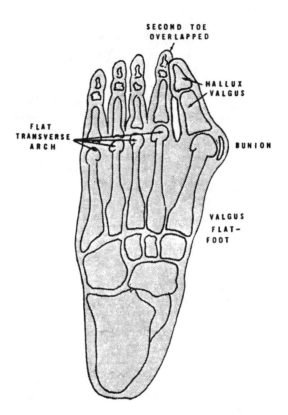

SECOND TOE
OVERLAPPED

HALLUX
VALGUS

FLAT
TRANSVERSE
ARCH

BUNION

VALGUS
FLAT-
FOOT

FIGURE 103. The foot with hallux valgus and bunion. The foot in which hallux valgus predominates is a broad forefoot with a depressed transverse metatarsal arch and a flattened longitudinal arch. The valgus big toe overrides or underlies the second toe, which may be secondarily a hammer toe. A swollen inflamed bursa may overlie the enlarged head of the first metatarsal.

If hallux valgus develops before the age of 20, there is usually a family history. In these cases, treatment should be conservative and consist of exercises with the wearing of a shoe modified to correct pes planus and pronation (see section on Treatment of the Pronated Foot in Chapter 5). A stabilizing splint may be worn at night (Fig. 105). A wide shoe with a flat heel should be worn by both girls and boys. A pounch may be pressed out or cut out at the site of the bunion. If surgery is indicated, the McBride procedure is preferred, as it immediately corrects the deformity and eliminates the tendency to recurrence by tendon transplants (Fig. 106). Following surgery, the patient must faithfully do corrective exercises and wear proper shoes.

132

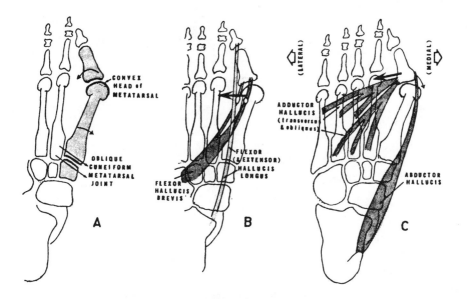

FIGURE 104. Concepts of hallux valgus causation. The most probable causes held responsible for hallux valgus are: *(A)* excessive convexity of the head of the first metatarsal that permits the phalanx to subluxate laterally. The oblique articular surface of the first cuneiform allows the metatarsal to angle medially to form *metatarsus varus primus*. *(B)* as the phalanges deviate laterally the flexor hallucis brevis and longus tendons on the plantar foot surface and the extensor hallucis longus on the dorsum act like a bowstring. *(C)* imbalance of the foot intrinsics in which the *ad*ductors over pull and shorten. The *ab*ductors are overpowered and elongate.

Hallux valgus in the elderly is best treated conservatively, including the use of molded shoes that prevent pressure being placed on the protruding portions of the foot. Correction of pronation in the fixed foot of the elderly should be done carefully as the deformities resist alteration. As the hallux valgus deformity of middle age is considered secondary to the strained flattened longitudinal arch and the concomitant splay foot with flattened transverse arch, restoration of these arches may afford relief. Exercise, arch supports, and corrective shoes should always precede surgical intervention. Discussion of the surgical procedures and their merits is beyond the scope of this book. However, two procedures are illustrated in Figure 106 as examples.

HALLUX RIGIDUS

Hallux rigidus is the second most common painful problem of the toes. Due to the inflexibility of the metatarsophalangeal joint of the big toe, the

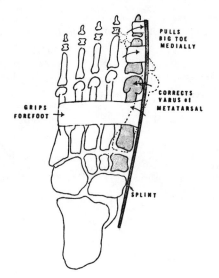

FIGURE 105. Night splint for juvenile hallux valgus.

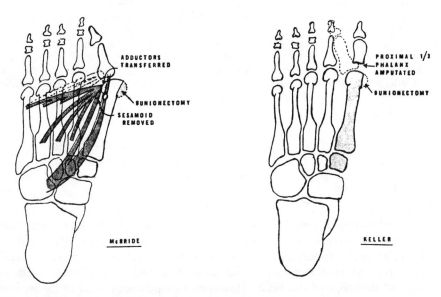

FIGURE 106. McBride and Keller operations for hallux valgus. The McBride operation consists of trimming the bunion, plicating the capsule on the medial aspect of the metatarsal head, and transplanting the adductor conjoined tendon from the base of the proximal phalanx to the outer head of the metatarsal. The adductor group now pulls the metatarsal laterally and does not subluxate the phalanx. The Keller operation trims the bunion and amputates the proximal one third of the proximal phalanx. The muscular attachments to the phalanx are removed. The sesamoids retract and the big toe shortens.

134

toe is unable to dorsiflex, which interferes with a smooth takeoff during gait. Every step normally requires dorsiflexion (extension) of the big toe, and impairment of motion at this joint may cause pain. A rigid toe that is asymptomatic does not require treatment. Only the partially rigid toe may be symptomatic, and once the fusion is complete, pain may disappear.

Diagnosis

Usually, the patient with hallux rigidus complains of pain elsewhere in the foot resulting from attempts to avoid big toe stress. The patient shifts weight to the outer border of the foot in order to prevent motion in the big toe. The foot is adducted and inverted to "roll-off" the head of the fifth metatarsal during walking. This is a tiring gait and pressure symptoms occur under the lateral metatarsal heads as well as at the first metatarsophalangeal joint which cannot be completely eliminated in walking.

Treatment

Hallux rigidus requires a shoe with a wide forefoot, which permits the forefoot to adduct, and one that is high enough to permit motion of the entire foot within it. A metatarsal pad placed under the first metatarsal and behind its head raises it and prevents dorsiflexion of the big toe. A metatarsal bar placed outside the shoe with an adequate rocker base aids the gait. A steel plate in the sole prevents flexion deformity of the shoe (Fig. 107). Surgery for hallux rigidus usually consists of resection of the joint and remodeling of the metatarsal head.

HAMMER TOE

Diagnosis

Hammer toe is a fixed flexion deformity of the interphalangeal joint. Any toe may be affected, but it is more prevalent in the second toe. In this condition, there is dorsiflexion of the proximal phalanx and flexion of the distal and middle phalanges (Fig. 108). The distal phalanx may point straight ahead but usually points downward. Calluses may form at its tip and also on the dorsum of the flexed interphalangeal joints from pressure against the shoe.

If the hammer toe is severe, the proximal phalanx will frequently sublux. The capsules and tendons on the flexed surfaces become contracted while on the opposite side they stretch. If there is a flexion deformity of only the distal phalanx, the condition is known as "mallet toe."

135

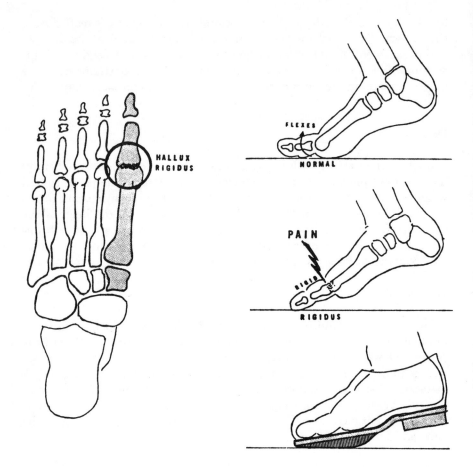

FIGURE 107. Hallux rigidus. Due to damage of the metatarsophalangeal joint, which becomes rigid, the toe will not flex on toe-off of the gait, and pain can occur at each step. Treatment consists of preventing stress on the rigid toe by placing a steel plate in the shoe sole to prevent bending and a rocker bar to permit pain-free gait.

Hammer toe is occasionally congenital, in which case it occurs in more than one toe and is associated with other congenital foot deformities. The acquired variety is the most common and usually occurs in a pronated foot. New shoes that are too short will often cause toes to hammer, as will tight elastic stockings of the wrong size. The second toe frequently becomes hammered in the hallux valgus as the big toe encroaches upon and under the second toe (see Fig. 103). Hammer toe may follow surgery performed for hallux valgus or hallux rigidus in which the flexor tendons are cut.

136

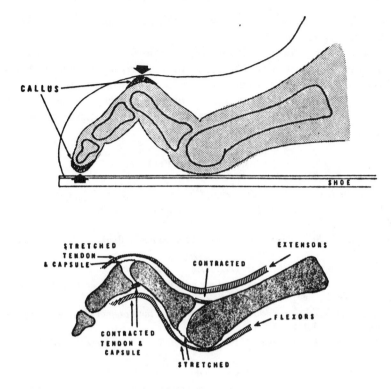

FIGURE 108. Hammer toe. The hammer toe is most often a flexion deformity of the interphalangeal joint, with the capsule and tendons contracted on the concave surface. Subluxation is frequent. The proximal phalanx is usually extended and the distal phalanx flexed and flexible. Pressure and friction result in painful calluses forming.

Treatment

In the treatment of hammer toe, it is important to avoid pressure over the protruding joints by the use of properly fitting shoes. The protruding joints may be protected by properly cut and fitted pads, or by bulging or cutting the shoe away from the potential callous site. The bulge in the shoe is made with a shoemaker's swan. The severely deformed foot may require custom-made "space shoes."

Manually stretching the contracted tissues of the flexed toes is seldom effective. When the deformity is disabling, surgery to fuse the toes in a straight position may be indicated. In the young, before changes become irreversible, tendon transplants are advocated. This consists of transplanting the flexor tendons to the extensor side of the toes. This procedure is feasible only in the middle three toes because transplanting tendons on the big toe will cause it to rotate and will result in a deformity as troublesome as the hammer toe.

Parents of very young children often express concern over a toe that overrides its neighbor. The fifth toe usually overrides the fourth. It is best to leave this condition untreated other than insuring proper shoes. If the condition becomes symptomatic, tenotomies and capsulotomies may be beneficial. The practice of amputating the fifth toe is usually rejected by the family.

BIBLIOGRAPHY

ADAMS, JC: *Outline of Orthopaedics,* ed 9. Churchill Livingston, New York, 1981.

BONNEY, G AND MACNAB, I: *Hallux valgus and hallux rigidus.* J Bone Joint Surg 34B:366, 1952.

CHOMELEY, JA: *Hallux valgus in adolescents.* Proceedings of the Royal Society of Medicine 51:903, 1958.

DUVRIES, HL: *Surgery of the Foot.* CV Mosby, St Louis, 1965.

GIBSON, J AND POGGOTT, H: *Osteotomy of the neck of the first metatarsal in the treatment of hallux valgus.* J Bone Joint Surg 44B:349, 1962.

KELIKIAN, H: *Hallux Valgus and Allied Deformities of the Forefoot and Metatarsalgia.* WB Saunders, Philadelphia, 1965, p 4.

KELLER, WL: *Surgical treatment of bunions and hallux valgus.* New York Medical Journal 80:741, 1904.

LAPIDUS, PW: *Operation for correction of hammer toe.* J Bone Joint Surg 21:4, 1939.

LEWIN, P: *The Foot and Ankle: Their Injuries, Diseases, Deformities, and Disabilities,* ed 4. Lea & Febiger, Philadelphia, 1959.

MCBRIDE, ED: *A conservative operation for bunions.* J Bone Joint Surg 10:735, 1928.

MIKHAIL, IK: *Bunion, hallux valgus, and metarsus primus varus.* Surg Gynecol Obstet 111:637, 1960.

MILGRAM, JE: *Office procedures for relief of the painful foot.* J Bone Joint Surg 46A:1095, 1964.

MITCHELL, CL, ET AL: *Osteotomy bunionectomy for hallux valgus.* J Bone Joint Surg 40A:4, 1958.

TAYLOR, RG: *The treatment of claw toes by multiple transfers of flexor into extensor tendons.* J Bone Joint Surg 33B:539, 1951.

WILSON, JN: *Oblique displacement osteotomy for hallux valgus.* J Bone Joint Surg 45B:552, 1963.

WILSON, JN: *The treatment of deformities of the foot and toes.* Br J Phy Med 17:73, 1954.

WILSON, JN: *V-Y correction for varus deformity of the fifth toe.* Br J Surg 41:133, 1953.

ZAMOSKY, I AND LICHT, S: *Shoes and their modifications.* In LICHT, S (ED): *Orthotics Etcetera, Physical Medicine Library,* Vol 9. Elizabeth Licht, Publisher, New Haven, 1966, p 388.

CHAPTER 9

Painful Conditions of the Heel

There are many varied reasons for a painful heel which can be classified under three headings: (1) pain arising in tissues behind and under the heel, (2) pain arising within the bones and joints of the heel, and (3) pain arising from a source not in the heel but referred there.

PLANTAR FASCIITIS

Pain felt *under the heel* is most frequently caused by a plantar fasciitis occurring with or without a "calcaneal spur." It is common in occupations that entail excessive standing or walking, especially when the patient has been unaccustomed to such activity. It is more common in a pronated foot, which has a flattened longitudinal arch, and frequently occurs after a period of bed rest. Men are more susceptible than women.

A bony prominence or spur may develop at the attachment of the plantar fascia to the calcaneus. This bony prominence may extend transversely across the entire plantar surface of the bone and is considered an ossification and calcification resulting from traction of the plantar fascia upon the periosteum, and occurs commonly without pain.

Pain and tenderness beneath the anterior portion of the heel often radiating into the sole is the presenting complaint. Examination reveals a point of deep tenderness at the anterior medial area of the calcaneus, the point of attachment of the plantar fascia (Fig. 109). X-ray films reveal nothing or a typical spur coming forward from the calcaneus. A spur is probably a coincidental finding, as they are often found in asymptomatic feet and often not found in patients with symptoms. The pain may be attributed to an infracalcaneal bursitis under the fascial attachment, to a traumatic periostitis, or the tearing of some of the fibers attaching to the bone.

Treatment is directed toward alleviating the pressure of weight bearing. Raising the heel ¼ inch removes the tension placed on the calcaneus

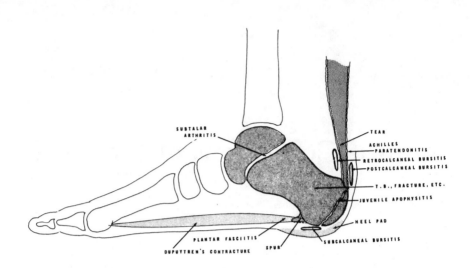

FIGURE 109. Sites of pain in the region of the heel.

by the Achilles tendon and releases the tension of the fascia by plantar flexing the forefoot. A sponge rubber cushion with its center removed may be placed under the heel, or a hole may be drilled into the sole of the shoe at the site of the heel and covered with sponge rubber.

Injections of cortisone and lidocaine (Novocain) into the painful region are effective. They may be injected directly into the area through the heel pad or by entering the heel from either the medial or lateral approach (Fig. 110). The injection is given at the site of maximum tenderness, and it is rarely necessary to give more than three weekly injections for relief. Any of the above measures may be used singly or in combination. It is rare that surgical removal of the spur and stripping of the plantar fascia from its posterior attachment must be resorted to. A high incidence of recurrence after surgery is claimed by many and denied by some.

PAINFUL HEEL PAD

Instead of localized pain as in plantar fasciitis, the pain may be generalized over the entire calcaneal pad. This pad is composed of fatty tissue and elastic fibrous tissue enclosed within compartments formed by fibrous septa. Young tissue has an elasticity which acts as a "shock absorber," but the elasticity decreases with age and the weight of the body must be borne by the unpadded calcaneus. This causes pain and if the condition is untreated, it results in scar formation and calcification of the calcaneus. Acute stress upon the pad may rupture or strain the compartments and cause temporary loss of compressibility.

140

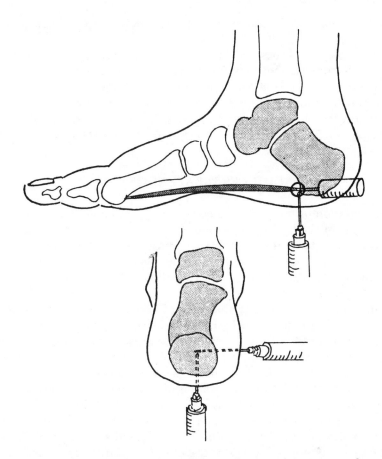

FIGURE 110. Injection technique in plantar fasciitis. The point of maximum tenderness of the plantar fascia can be injected directly through the heel pad. This is the area where the fascia inserts into the calcaneus. The site can be reached from the lateral or medial approach but localization by this approach is less accurate.

The usual painful heel pad is self-limited and responds to relieving the pressure either by inserting a sponge rubber heel pad, as described in treatment of the spur, or by raising the heel to transfer the weight anteriorly. Infiltration of 5 to 10 ml of lidocaine (Novocain) under the pad may relieve the symptoms.

DUPUYTREN'S CONTRACTURE

Dupuytren's contracture, similar to that found in the palm, may occur in the plantar fascia (see Fig. 109). This condition presents lobulated firm nodules that appear to coalesce within the plantar fascia. They usually

141

occur in middle age and apparently occur more frequently in patients with epilepsy.

The tumors are fibrous and biopsy reveals cellular components of proliferating fibroblasts that may be confused with fibrosarcoma. They are adherent to the skin but show no signs of inflammation. They grow slowly and their symptoms are those of a mechanical nature. Treatment consists of excision of the entire mass and the involved fascia. As in the similar palmar lesions, recurrences are frequent but the condition is benign.

ACHILLES PARATENDONITIS

Inflammation of the paratendonous tissues may cause pain on the posterior aspect of the heel in the region of the Achilles tendon insertion (see Fig. 109). The term tenosynovitis is a misnomer when applied to this condition, as the Achilles tendon has no synovial tendon sheath. The inflammation occurs in the loose connective tissue about the tendon known as paratenon.

Trauma or stress is usually the cause. There is generalized tenderness when the tendon is squeezed by the examiner's fingers. The tendon usually appears normal but there may be some thickening. Occasionally, it is swollen, distended, and exhibits crepitation during motion. Running, jumping, or dancing, which stretches the Achilles tendon, causes pain.

Treatment consists of immobilization of the ankle in a below-the-knee plaster cast for four weeks. Cortisone injected deep to the tendon may be beneficial. This injection may enter the inflamed retrocalcaneal bursa, which may be the cause of the painful Achilles tendon. Surgical excision of the inflamed connective tissues or the inflamed bursa may be needed.

POSTERIOR CALCANEAL BURSITIS

Pain and tenderness of the posterior aspect of the heel and under the skin occurring especially in women is due to a postcalcaneal bursitis, which is inflammation of the bursa located between the Achilles tendon and the skin (see Fig. 109). This condition is usually caused by friction from ill-fitting shoes and is prevalent in women who wear high-heeled shoes. The bursa is usually visibly inflamed and often distended with fluid. Chronic irritation will thicken the walls of the bursa and the overlying skin.

Examination reveals an inflamed and thickened area at the back of the heel where the upper margin of the shoe rubs, and tenderness and swelling are easily detected. Treatment begins with properly fitted shoes with moderately low heels. Moleskin placed over the thickened skin prevents further friction. The backs of the shoes may have to be cut out or the heel raised inside the shoe. Surgical excision of the bursa is never indicated. Drainage of the swollen bursa may be done by needle aspiration followed by the insertion of hydrocortisone into the sac.

CALCANEAL APOPHYSITIS

Calcaneal apophysitis, also called Sever's disease, is a painful condition occurring in adolescents. Most prevalent in active adolescent boys between the ages of 8 and 13 years, it is the result of an acute or chronic strain of the Achilles tendon on the posterior apophysis of the calcaneus that has not yet fused. It has been classified among the general osteochondrosis syndromes, which include Legg-Calvé-Perthes disease of the hip and Osgood-Schlatter disease of the tibial tuberosity and can be considered a traction injury.

A diagnosis of apophysitis is suggested when a teen-ager complains of pain and sensitivity at the back of the heel below the attachment of the Achilles tendon. The condition is often bilateral. Walking may be completely without pain, and often the only complaint is tenderness to touch or pressure. As wearing shoes may cause pain, there may be some swelling in the area. The pain is aggravated by standing on tiptoes or running.

X-ray examination is usually of no assistance in diagnosis. The noted "fragmentation" of the apophysis does not significantly differ from that of the normal heel at that age, but unilateral fragmentation with bony condensation of the epiphysis does supplement the clinical picture and confirm the diagnosis.

Treatment is symptomatic. The condition is self-limited, and symptoms usually subside spontaneously. Efforts should be made to curtail the physical activities of the child to within the limits of pain, until symptoms subside. This presents a problem in active adolescents as symptoms may persist for many months if trauma continues. A shoe heel built up 1/4 inch places the foot in equinus and lessens the strain of the Achilles at its insertion. Crutches may be beneficial when the condition is unilateral. In severe cases, the leg is placed in a plaster cast extending above the knee; the knee is flexed and the foot placed in equinus. The prognosis of ultimate recovery without residual disability allays parental concern when pain and tenderness persist.

RUPTURED ACHILLES TENDON

A partial or complete rupture of the Achilles tendon may occur at the narrowest portion of the tendon some 2 inches above its point of attachment. It occurs most often in men 40 to 50 years old and has its highest incidence in men with normally sedentary habits who suddenly engage in more strenuous activities.

Rupture of the Achilles tendon occurs in several manners: (1) an extra stretch to a fully stretched tendon, (2) forceful ankle dorsiflexion when the ankle is relaxed and unprepared, or (3) direct trauma to the tendon while it is taut.

The major complaint is acute agonizing pain felt in the lower calf, which makes walking impossible. The patient's feet are examined while the patient is kneeling on a table with both feet hanging over the edge. In this position, the affected foot is less plantar flexed than the other if rupture is complete. A gap in the Achilles tendon can often be palpated and the belly of the gastrocnemius is retracted into the upper calf (Fig. 111). If rupture is complete, the ankle can be dorsiflexed to a greater degree than normal, but if the rupture is partial, dorsiflexion is not increased. The *Simmond's test* consists of squeezing the calf while patient is lying prone with both feet over the edge of the examining table. In the normal ankle, gastroc-plantar flexion will occur, but in the complete tendon tear the ankle will not move. The patient who has sustained a complete tear cannot rise on tiptoes. Ecchymoses are found around the heel.

Partial tears usually become complete at a later date. This later tear may be painless with the patient merely experiencing a sudden fall to the ground as the leg "gives out" as if the patient had been tripped. Examination will confirm the complete tear.

One school of thought stated that patients with ruptures of the Achilles tendon should undergo surgery without delay. This was refuted in the early 1970s, when nonsurgical treatment was advocated with claims of equal or greater success.

Surgical treatment employs suturing of the tendon and the paratenon with heavy suture material. Postoperatively, a below-the-knee plaster cast of the foot in slight equinus is indicated for approximately seven weeks (range, six to nine weeks). Nonsurgical treatment requires a below-the-knee plaster cast with foot in gravity plantar flexion for four weeks, then recasting with less equinus but permitting cast ambulation. Total casting is advocated for approximately eight weeks (range, seven to nine weeks). Upon removal of the cast, a 2.5 centimeter heel is worn for ambulation for four weeks, or until the ankle can be dorsiflexed 10°.

Comparison of the surgical versus the nonsurgical treatment reports only minor differences in results with the advantage of the nonsurgical having a lower morbidity and no hospitalization. The incidence of restricted activities and rerupture did not advocate open- versus closed-reduction repair.

SUBTALAR ARTHRITIS

Pain that is felt *within the heel* may be *referred* from an arthritic subtalar joint (see Fig. 109). Arthritis of this joint frequently follows

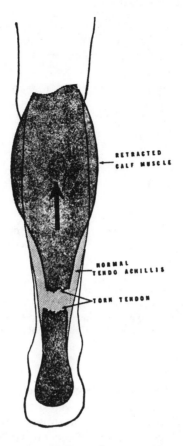

FIGURE 111. Torn Achilles tendon. Most Achilles tendon tears are complete and occur approximately two inches above the calcaneal insert. The calf muscle retracts toward the popliteal space and a "gap" often can be felt at the site of the tear. Patient cannot rise on tiptoes.

trauma, such as a fracture of the calcaneus. Pain is felt on motion of the subtalar joint, and x-ray examination reveals irregularity of the bones between the talus and the calcaneus. Crepitation may be elicited by this motion, and tenderness may be elicited from pressure over the sinus tarsi in front of the lateral malleolus. Muscle spasm, especially of the peroneal group, may exist in an attempt to splint the subtalar joint. Weight bearing is painful and rest affords relief. Conservative treatment is usually satisfactory but surgical fusion may be necessary if symptoms warrant.

FRACTURES

A fracture must always be suspected when pain in the heel occurs after trauma. Fracture of the calcaneus may result whenever a falling person

145

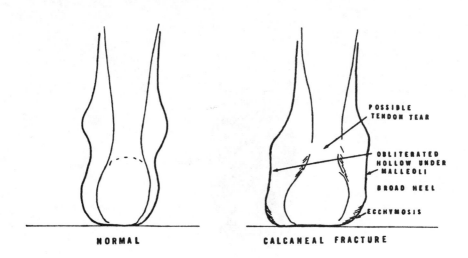

POSSIBLE
TENDON TEAR

OBLITERATED
HOLLOW UNDER
MALLEOLI

BROAD HEEL

ECCHYMOSIS

NORMAL   CALCANEAL FRACTURE

FIGURE 112. Fracture of the calcaneus. A fracture of the calcaneus is suspect when there is a history of trauma and the heel appears broad, the hollows below the malleoli are obliterated, and there is ecchymosis in the plantar surface of the heel. Motion is restricted in attempting inversion and eversion of the calcaneus. Gait is painful. X-ray examination confirms the diagnosis.

lands on the feet. Characteristic signs suggest a fracture (Fig. 112). The heel is broadened, and the hollows beneath the malleoli are obliterated because of exudate. Ecchymosis later appears around the heel. All movements of the calcaneus are painful and markedly restricted. X-ray films must be taken to confirm the presence, site, and extent of the fracture.

Fractures of the calcaneus result in prolonged incapacity and in some cases permanent disability and pain. A fracture of the calcaneus may be accompanied by a compression fracture of a vertebra or avulsion of the Achilles tendon from its insertion. These must be kept in mind when dealing with a fractured calcaneus. The treatment of calcaneal fractures is beyond the scope of this book and the reader is referred to the literature on the subject.

REFERRED PAIN

Pain can be referred to the region of the heel from entrapment of the posterior tibial nerve and its calcaneal branch. This condition is fully discussed in Chapter 11 and depicted in Figure 125. Pain may be referred to the region of the heel from irritation of the S_1 nerve root in lumbar diskogenic disease (see Fig. 130). For no known reason, pain in the heel is a frequent complaint in a patient with early rheumatoid spondylitis.

BIBLIOGRAPHY

ADAMS, JC: *Outline of Orthopaedics,* ed 9. Churchill Livingston, New York, 1981.

DuVRIES, HL: *Surgery of the Foot.* CV Mosby, St Louis, 1965.

GROSS, D: *Ankylosing Spondylitis.* Folia Rheumat 1, Documenta Geigy, Basel, Switzerland, 1965.

HOOKER, CH: *Rupture of the tendo calcaneus.* J Bone Joint Surg 45-B:360, 1963.

LINDHOLM, A: *A New method of operation in subcutaneous rupture of the Achilles tendon.* Acta Chir Scand 117:261, 1959.

MEYERDING, H AND SHELLITO, JG: *Dupuytren's contracture of the foot.* Journal of the International College of Surgery 11:596, 1948.

MOSELEY, HF: *Traumatic disorders of the ankle and foot.* Clin Symp 17-3:30, 1965.

NISTOR, L: *Surgical and nonsurgical treatment of Achilles tendon rupture: A prospective randomized study.* J Bone Joint Surg 63-A:394, 1981.

NISTOR, L: *Conservative treatment of fresh subcutaneous rupture of the Achilles tendon.* Acta Orthop Scand 47:459, 1976.

PERSSON, A AND WREDMARK, T: *The Treatment of total ruptures of the Achilles tendon by plantar immobilization.* Int Orthop 3:149, 1979.

SHIELDS, PL, ET AL: *The Cybex II evaluation of surgically repaired Achilles tendon ruptures.* Am J Sports Med 6:369, 1978.

TUREK, SL: *Orthopaedics: Principles and Their Application,* ed 3. JB Lippincott, Philadelphia, 1977.

WATSON-JONES, R: *Fractures and Joint Injuries,* ed 4. Williams & Wilkins, Baltimore, 1955.

WILSON, JN: *The Treatment of deformities of the foot and toes.* Br J Phys Med 17:73, 1954.

ZADEK, I: *Repair of old rupture of the tendo Achilles by means of fascialata.* J Bone Joint Surg 22:1070, 1940.

CHAPTER 10

Injuries to the Ankle

The sprained ankle is the most common injury that causes pain in the ankle. This condition varies from a simple strain of the ligaments to tearing of the ligaments with or without avulsion of the bones to which they attach. The most severe injury is the fracture-dislocation. The unwary physician who diagnoses every injury to the ankle as a "mere sprain" is harboring a false sense of security and denying proper treatment to the patient. The statement of Watson-Jones that "it is worse to sprain an ankle than to break it" has foundation if every sprain receives the same diagnosis and treatment.

The ankle joint is between the talus, tibia, and fibula and is stable because of its mechanical configuration and ligamentous supports (see Figs. 3 and 4). The talus has no muscles attached to it, fits snugly between the two malleoli, and is directly aligned below the tibia. In the dorsiflexed position the broader aspect of the talus is forced between the malleoli, and no lateral motion is permitted. In the plantar flexed position the narrow portion of the talus presents itself between the malleoli and some lateral motion is possible (see Fig. 5). The neutral position and especially the plantar flexed position therefore lend themselves to the possibility of a sprain most often.

The lateral and medial collateral ligaments stabilize the ankle joint, yet permit plantar flexion and dorsiflexion (see Fig. 6). The medial ligaments have an eccentric axis of rotation (see Fig. 7) so that all are taut in the neutral position, but the posterior strands relax in plantar flexion and the anterior fibers relax in dorsiflexion. The lateral collateral ligaments have a central axis and remain taut in all ranges of plantar flexion or dorsiflexion.

EXTERNAL COLLATERAL LIGAMENT. This ligament consists of three distinct bands (Fig. 113):

1. Anterior talofibular ligament: passes from the tip of the fibula to the base of the neck of the talus on its lateral aspect.

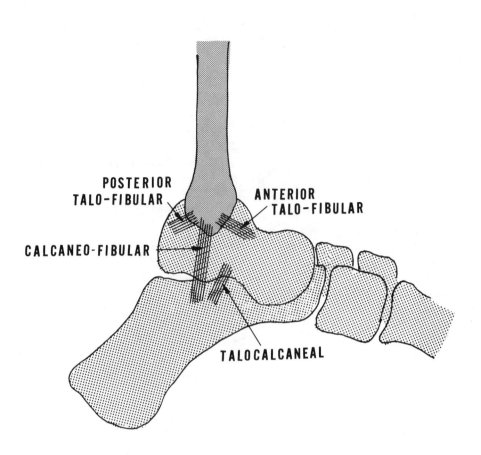

POSTERIOR
TALO-FIBULAR

ANTERIOR
TALO-FIBULAR

CALCANEO-FIBULAR

TALOCALCANEAL

FIGURE 113. Lateral collateral ligament.

2. Calcaneofibular ligament: extends down from the fibula and slightly
   posterior to the calcaneus.
3. Posterior talofibular ligament: passes backward horizontally and inserts on the tubercle of the talus.

The external collateral ligament is the most frequently involved in soft
tissue injury to the ankle. Forceful inversion damages the anterior talofibular and the calcaneofibular ligaments with tearing, mostly at their
fibular attachment or by avulsion of the fibula tip. In case of injury,
excessive inversion results and dependent on whether the anterior or the
posterior talofibular ligament is torn, a positive "drawer sign" (shear motion) can be elicited.

INTERNAL COLLATERAL LIGAMENT. The internal collateral ligament is
termed the deltoid ligament and is formed by four branches coursing
from the internal malleolus of the ankle mortise (Fig. 114):

149

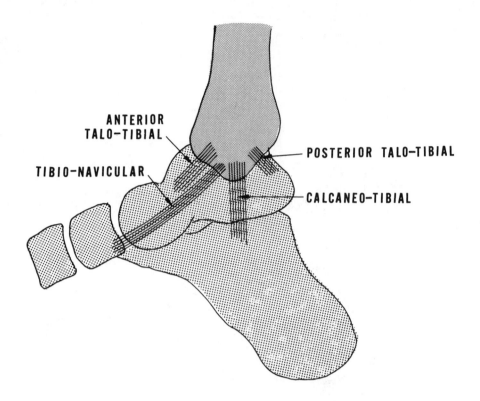

ANTERIOR
TALO-TIBIAL

POSTERIOR TALO-TIBIAL

TIBIO-NAVICULAR

CALCANEO-TIBIAL

FIGURE 114. Medial (deltoid) collateral ligament.

1. Tibio-navicular band.
2. Anterior talo-tibial.
3. Calcaneo-tibial.
4. Posterior talo-tibial.

The ligaments are supplied with sensory nerves which, when stretched, invoke a reflex muscle spasm which protects the joint from further motion.

The ankle is most unstable when plantar flexed, and it is in this position that forceful inversion or eversion will stretch the ligaments. This action can occur when running, walking over uneven ground, in athletic activities, or even from unaccustomed walking in high-heeled shoes.

A "sprain" may be defined as a rupture of some or all of the fibers of a ligament. A sprain is considered *minor* when the number of ruptured fibers do not cause instability of the joint. A *major* sprain has sufficient numbers of fibers torn to result in joint instability. With a minor ankle ligament sprain, inversion and eversion range of motion does not exceed

150

normal whereas it does in major sprains. A positive "drawer sign" occurs in a major sprain.

INVERSION SPRAINS

The most common sprain occurs from inversion stress when the foot is slightly plantar flexed and results in stretch of the lateral collateral ligaments. The anterior talofibular ligament is the most commonly affected. If the inversion stress occurs with the ankle at right angle, the calcaneofibular ligament receives the stretch force.

Strain is merely an overstretching of the ligament without disruption of the integrity of its fibers or avulsion from its bony attachment. This may be considered a minor injury and recovery occurs within a few weeks. If the stress is more severe, the fibers may tear and a severe *sprain* has occurred. The ligament rarely tears in its middle, but sustains a tear at its proximal or distal point of attachment. A small fragment of bone may be avulsed with the ligament rather than the ligament itself being torn.

The simple strain retains normal joint stability, whereas the severe sprain with tear of the ligament or avulsion of its bony attachment results in instability. The ankle joint dislocates. The degree of dislocation termed *subluxation* implies partial separation of the bones with large areas remaining in contact, whereas *dislocation* connotes complete separation of the adjacent bones. The differentiation of simple strain from a sprain with some degree of dislocation is suspected clinically and verified by x-ray examination.

Diagnosis

The diagnosis of the injury is best made at the site of the accident when the patient has a clear recollection of the manner of injury. Later, the details become vague and the site of pain is less localized. The subsequent swelling and ecchymosis also are less specific at a later date. The history given by the patient or a bystander will reveal the ankle motion that caused the injury and the site of immediate pain and tenderness. There may have been an audible "snap" or a sensation of "tearing."

In the simple strain, if the foot is passively inverted, the talus remains in its proper position and no gap can be palpated between it and the malleolus. Protective spasm may deceive the examiner in the early phase, therefore, any severe sprain should be considered to be a potential tear or avulsion until confirmed or denied by x-ray examination. If a tear has occurred, the foot can be inverted to a greater degree than normal and the talus separates from the lateral malleolus. A palpable sulcus may permit insertion of a fingertip between the talus and the lateral malleolus.

151

X-ray films taken with the foot inverted will reveal abnormal tilt of the talus within the mortise (Fig. 115).

All patients with significant ankle injuries should have an x-ray examination. To reveal tilting of the talus within the mortise, which normally is insignificant, the ankle must be fully inverted, then x-ray photographs taken in this position. The practice of injecting lidocaine (Novocain) into the area of ligamentous strain to "overcome" the pain and spasm is usually unnecessary if the ankle is moved gently and slowly. The degree of talar tilt indicates the presence and extent of a tear of the ligaments.

With a sprain, there will ultimately be an effusion into the ankle joint that will distend the joint and cause the foot to invert and dorsiflex. The swelling is first noted beneath the extensor tendons, usually anterior to the lateral malleolus, and eventually will be seen on either side of the Achilles tendon behind the malleoli. Ecchymosis may occur indicating injury to blood vessels in the area.

The range of plantar flexion and dorsiflexion of the ankle joint may remain normal in spite of severe lateral ligamentous tear. Normally inversion and eversion are markedly limited or nonexistent in the dorsiflexed joint, so any such motion that occurs with the foot dorsiflexed indicates ligamentous laxity or tear. To test this motion, the calcaneus must be grasped and motion attempted there. A false impression will be received if the forefoot rather than the calcaneus is moved. *Testing for excessive*

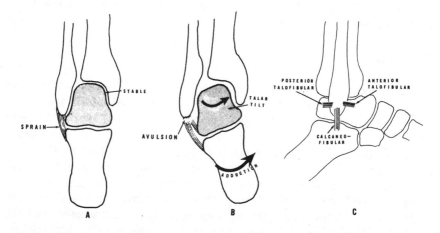

FIGURE 115. Lateral ligamentous sprain and avulsion. The lateral ligaments of the ankle are depicted in *C*. The anterior talofibular and the calcaneofibular ligaments are the ligaments most frequently involved in inversion injuries. *A* is the simple sprain in which the ligaments remain intact and the talus remains stable within the mortise. *B* depicts avulsion of the lateral ligaments, and the talus becomes unstable and *tilts* within the mortise when the calcaneus is adducted.

152

range of motion should not delay the institution of appropriate treatment. Specific treatment after establishing a more precise diagnosis will be possible and more effective if immediate care is instituted regardless of the severity of the injury.

Treatment

Control of swelling is the immediate consideration. Effusion and hemorrhage distend the joint and overstretch the ligaments. The presence of effusion also favors the formation of adhesions which delay healing. Swelling can be minimized by (1) the immediate application of a firm bandage, (2) the application of cold, and (3) elevation of the leg. Bandaging must be firm and must include the entire foot from behind the toes to the lower half of the leg. Two inch gauze, crepe bandage, or an elastic bandage may be used. Adhesive tape is permissible but less desirable because it may be irritating to the skin and difficult to remove.

The bandaged ankle should be placed in cold or ice water immediately. If this is not feasible, ice packs around the elevated foot may be used. The duration of immersion is arbitrary and varies with the severity of the injury. As a rule 15 to 20 minutes of immersion, followed by elevation of the leg, repeated every 3 to 6 hours, will suffice. Oral phenylbutazone may be used in the hope of minimizing inflammation.

X-ray films should be taken as soon as possible, especially if fracture is suspected. Routine films through the bandage will reveal the more obvious fractures. If avulsion of the ligaments is suspected, as it should in all severe injuries, "stress" films should be taken. The attending physician should hold the foot in marked inversion while the films are taken to insure that proper views are obtained.

If only a strain is diagnosed, the foot may be rebandaged daily and ice packs continued for several more days. After three or four days the ice packs are replaced by hot soaks. The bandage should not be removed too soon or the swelling may return. Usually, after 7 to 10 days the bandage can be removed safely.

Non-weight-bearing exercises should be started within the first few days. They should be done actively by the patient and not forcefully by a therapist or a relative. The foot should be moved through full range of motion: full plantar flexion, dorsiflexion, inversion, eversion, and toe flexion. These motions, done frequently during the day, will help disperse the edema and avoid the formation of adhesions as well as maintain muscle tone. Hot and cold contrast baths, whirlpool, ultrasound therapy, and iontophoresis, if available, may hasten recovery, but are not superior to heat and active exercises.

When the swelling has significantly subsided or disappeared, and the ankle has been proven to have no ligamentous tear, the ankle should be taped in a basket-weave fashion (Fig. 116) and weight bearing resumed. Competitive sports should be avoided for at least one to three weeks depending on the appearance, function, and pain of the ankle. If discomfort persists, and the patient feels insecure in spite of the ankle appearing stable in clinical examination and stress films, a lateral wedge may be added to the heel of the shoe (Fig. 117). Taping of the ankle should be continued for several weeks.

Treatment of the inversion injury with avulsion or tear of the lateral ligament must be energetic. A plaster cast is applied holding the foot at a right angle to the leg with the foot and ankle in slight *eversion*. The cast is applied even in the presence of swelling and is removed and replaced as the swelling decreases and the cast becomes loose fitting. The cast should be kept on for 10 weeks and may include a walking heel.

Some favor surgical repair of completely avulsed ligaments, but it is generally accepted that an ankle properly immobilized for a sufficient length of time will heal satisfactorily. After removal of the cast, active exercises should be initiated in order to regain range of motion and strength of the foot and ankle muscles. The proprioceptive sense of the ligaments and muscles must be retrained by coordination and balancing exercises.

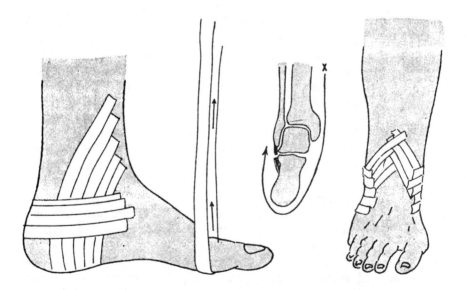

FIGURE 116. Taping a sprained ankle. The purpose of taping an ankle is to prevent further stretching of the injured ligaments until healing has occurred. The ankle must be inverted or everted to place the strained ligament at rest. The center figure depicts an avulsed lateral ligament. The tape here begins from inside and runs under the foot to finish on the outer leg holding the heel *everted*. The horizontal strips minimize rotation of the forefoot.

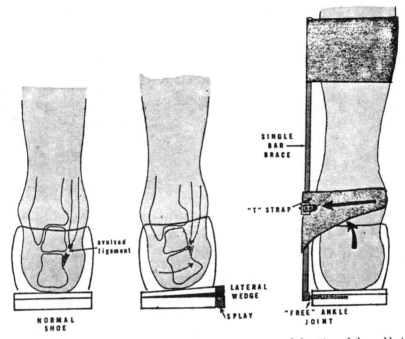

FIGURE 117. Conservative treatment of the chronic recurrent dislocation of the ankle joint. When the lateral ligaments are avulsed and improperly treated, the ankle becomes unstable. A lateral heel and sole wedge plus a splay heel maintains the foot in an everted position. An inside single bar brace with an inside pulling "T" strap maintains eversion.

"Chronic sprain" or recurrent dislocations usually imply improper treatment of the initial acute injury. Treatment of these recurring sprains must include support of the ankle. This is done by using an outside heel and sole wedge, a "splay" heel on the shoe, a brace with a "T" strap pulling the ankle toward the inside upright bar, exercises to strengthen the evertor muscles of the foot and ankle, and exercises to improve balance coordination. Persistence of disability will often require surgical intervention.

EVERSION SPRAINS

An injury to the ankle that forcefully *everts* the ankle will usually cause bony damage rather than straining or tearing of the medial ligament alone as in the *inversion* type of injury. The more frequent ankle injury, forceful inversion, causes mostly ligamentous injury and only rarely involves bone. In an eversion injury the medial ligament is so strong that fracture or avulsion of the tibia will occur before the ligament tears. Although tearing of the deltoid ligament is infrequent it must be con-

155

stantly suspected to prevent the serious consequences of improper treatment.

Tibiofibular Ligament Tear

A sprain of the medial ligaments may tear the inferior tibiofibular ligament. This ligamentous tear permits the ankle mortise to widen and causes an unstable ankle joint. The talus is allowed lateral motion within the mortise which ultimately leads to degenerative changes of the joint (Fig. 118).

Diagnosis

Widening of the ankle mortise can easily be missed clinically. The tear of the tibiofibular ligament and the separation of the malleoli must be suspected and confirmed by x-ray examination. The pathognomonic sign on the x-ray film is a widening of the joint space between the medial border of the talus and the medial malleolus (Fig. 118C). Routine

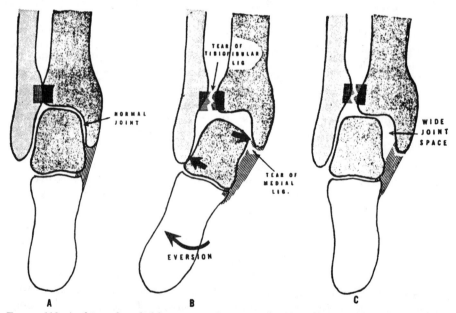

FIGURE 118. Avulsion of medial ligament and anterior tibiofibular ligaments from eversion injury to the ankle. A depicts the normal ankle mortise with the talus snugly between the malleoli. The eversion stress separates the malleoli (arrows), tears the anterior tibiofibular ligaments and the medial deltoid ligaments (B). Once the ankle has returned to its neutral position (C) a wide space remains between the talus and the medial malleolus which is a diagnostic sign on x-ray films. With the wide mortise, the ankle remains unstable.

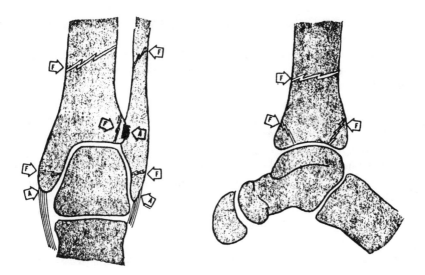

FIGURE 119. Sites of fracture and ligamentous avulsion. Fractures can occur at all the depicted sites. These fractures can be single, in combination, with or without ligamentous tear or avulsion, or with any combination of dislocation. *F* indicates fracture, *A* avulsion of ligament. Proper diagnosis is by x-ray examination.

ankle views may fail to reveal this separation, as the lower tibia and fibula frequently overlap on a direct anterior-posterior view. An oblique view when compared with a similar view of the other ankle will often reveal the separation.

Treatment

Treatment of the torn deltoid and inferior tibiofibular ligaments attempts approximating the two malleoli in order to reform the mortise and seat the talus snugly. This is done by plaster casting with the ankle compressed bilaterally. After 10 days, or sooner if the swelling has subsided and the cast has loosened, a new cast is applied. After three to six weeks a third cast is applied to further compress the malleoli together. No weight bearing is permitted for eight weeks.

Internal fixation with a screw inserted between the tibia and the fibula may be necessary to reduce the separation and approximate the two fragments. Many feel this procedure is always indicated, but *internal fixation with a screw does not permit earlier weight bearing, nor does it eliminate the need for plaster casting.* The screw merely assures anatomic reduction and immobilization within the cast. It presents all the adverse effects of open reduction as opposed to closed reduction.

157

FRACTURES AND FRACTURE DISLOCATIONS

Treatment of fractures and fracture dislocations is beyond the scope of this book. Fractures and fracture dislocations result from stresses similar to those that cause ligamentous injuries, which reaffirms the need for x-ray studies of the injured ankle. Initial treatment of the injured ankle with a possible fracture is as for the severe sprain and involves careful handling to attempt gentle correction of the gross deformity to prevent compounding the fracture and impairing the circulation. Splinting for transportation, elevation of the leg, application of cold, and firm dressing will minimize the swelling without impairment of circulation. The particular fracture must then receive its specific treatment (Fig. 119).

BIBLIOGRAPHY

CLAYTON, ML AND WEIR, GJ: *Experimental investigations of ligamentous healing.* Am J Surg 98:373, 1959.

DePALMA, AF: *Section I, symposium: Injuries to the ankle joint.* Clin Orthop 42:2, 1965.

DuVRIES, HL: *Surgery of the Foot.* CV Mosby, St Louis, 1965.

FREEMAN, MAR, DEAN, MRE, AND HANHAM, IWF: *The etiology and prevention of functional instability of the foot.* J Bone Joint Surg 47-B:678.

GRIFFITHS, JC: *Tendon injuries around the ankle.* J Bone Joint Surg 47-B:686.

KAPLAN, E: *Some principles of anatomy and kinesiology in stabilizing operations of the foot.* Clin Orthop 34:7, 1964.

LEWIN, P: *The Foot and Ankle,* ed 4. Lea & Febiger, Philadelphia, 1959.

McLAUGHTON, HL: *Trauma.* WB Saunders, Philadelphia, 1959.

MOSELY, HF: *Traumatic disorders of the ankle and foot.* Clin Sympos 17-3:30, 1965.

RUBIN, G AND WITTEN, M: *The talar tilt angle and the fibular collateral ligaments.* J Bone Joint Surg 42-A:311, 1960.

CHAPTER 11

Neurologic Disorders of the Foot

Foot disturbances attributable to nerve involvement are rarely due to intrinsic causes in the foot proper. Most neurologic disorders of the foot are caused by impairment of nerves proximal to it, involving either a peripheral nerve or some portion of the central nervous system.

INNERVATION OF THE FOOT

The foot and ankle are innervated by spinal segments of L_4, L_5, S_1, and S_2. These segments descend the posterior thigh in the sciatic nerve and ultimately divide into the tibial and the peroneal nerves (see Fig. 26) which supply the musculature of the foot and ankle. The muscles that plantar flex the foot and ankle are innervated by the tibial nerve, those that dorsiflex by the deep peroneal branch of the common peroneal nerve, and those that evert by the superficial branch of the common peroneal nerves. The small plantar muscles receive their innervation from the distal branches of the posterior tibial nerve after it has reached the sole of the foot and divided into the lateral and medial plantar nerves.

If the sciatic nerve is severed, total paralysis of all the muscles below the knee will result, together with loss of sensation on the outer side of the leg and almost the entire foot. A small area on the inner surface of the heel will be spared loss of sensation.

The sensory pattern of the peripheral nerves of the leg has been shown previously in Figure 27. The combination of specific motor weakness with hypalgesia of skin surfaces will reveal which nerve or nerves are impaired.

Injury to the deep peroneal nerve impairs dorsiflexion of the foot and toes and causes a drop foot resulting in a steppage gait. Hypalgesia is confined to a small area of the dorsum of the foot between the first and second toes. Because the superficial peroneal nerve remains intact, the foot everts during gait resulting in a valgus foot.

159

Injury to the superficial peroneal nerve paralyzes the evertors of the foot causing inversion with an ultimate equinovarus foot position. The anterior lateral aspect of the leg and the dorsum of the foot lose sensation. Injury to the common peroneal nerve combines the motor and sensory losses just described for the deep and superficial nerves. The foot is now "dropped" and has some inversion due to the unopposed action of the posterior tibial muscle.

Because the plantar and toe flexors are innervated by the tibial nerve, the patient is unable to rise on tiptoes or to flex the toes when this nerve is damaged. There is sensory loss on the plantar surface of the foot with ultimate atrophy of the calf and the intrinsic muscles of the foot. The exact level of nerve injury will determine the extent of motor loss and vice versa.

Determining whether a motor impairment is at (1) the anterior horn cell level, (2) the root level (Fig. 120), (3) the spinal nerve level, or (4) the peripheral nerve level may pose some difficulty. Figure 121 depicts the components leading to the formation of a peripheral nerve and specific muscle innervation. Localization of the site of nerve impairment is possi-

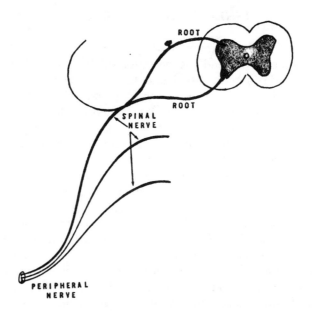

FIGURE 120. Formation of a peripheral nerve. A sensory and motor root emerge from the spinal cord. They merge to form a spinal segmental nerve. The area served by the sensory portion of this nerve is called a dermatome. The muscles innervated by the motor segment are a myotome. Several segmental nerves may merge to form a peripheral nerve which is both sensory and motor.

160

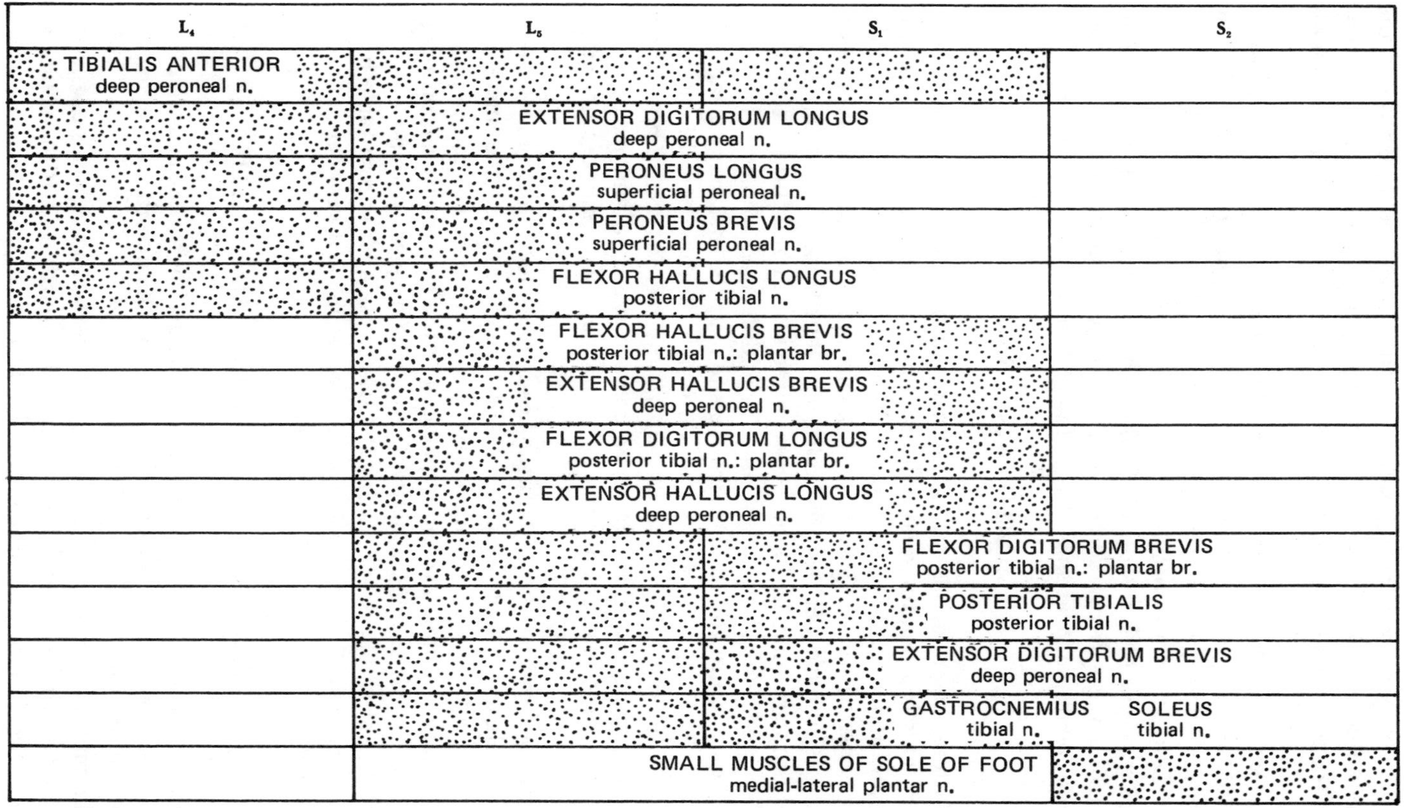

Chart — Origin of nerve roots in spinal segments (columns: L_4, L_5, S_1, S_2)

- TIBIALIS ANTERIOR — deep peroneal n.
- EXTENSOR DIGITORUM LONGUS — deep peroneal n.
- PERONEUS LONGUS — superficial peroneal n.
- PERONEUS BREVIS — superficial peroneal n.
- FLEXOR HALLUCIS LONGUS — posterior tibial n.
- FLEXOR HALLUCIS BREVIS — posterior tibial n.: plantar br.
- EXTENSOR HALLUCIS BREVIS — deep peroneal n.
- FLEXOR DIGITORUM LONGUS — posterior tibial n.: plantar br.
- EXTENSOR HALLUCIS LONGUS — deep peroneal n.
- FLEXOR DIGITORUM BREVIS — posterior tibial n.: plantar br.
- POSTERIOR TIBIALIS — posterior tibial n.
- EXTENSOR DIGITORUM BREVIS — deep peroneal n.
- GASTROCNEMIUS — tibial n.
- SOLEUS — tibial n.
- SMALL MUSCLES OF SOLE OF FOOT — medial-lateral plantar n.

FIGURE 121. Origin of nerve roots in spinal segments. Chart shows innervation of the muscles involved in gait and the gray area the spinal segments of origin.

ble by manual muscle testing, sensory pattern mapping, and electromyographic testing. More recently, nerve conduction determination has entered the field of neuromuscular diagnosis making diagnosis and prognosis more accurate.

The function of any nerve along its path may be impaired by mechanical irritation or compression resulting in an entrapment neuropathy. Here motor and sensory loss and pain may result, with the pain usually present at rest and sometimes becoming severe at night. The nerve distal to the site of entrapment is frequently tender. The pain may confuse the examiner by having a retrograde distribution, thus causing suspicion of a peripheral neuropathy arising at a different level.

MORTON'S NEURALGIA

Morton's neuralgia is an entrapment neuropathy of an interdigital nerve. This is a painful condition resulting from a neoplasm, a fusiform swelling about 3/4 inch long, on a digital nerve. It is most commonly found where the interdigital nerve branches into the contiguous aspects of the digits, usually between the third and fourth toes (Fig. 122). An unusual neoplasm may be found between the second and third metatarsals.

This condition is found most often in middle-aged women. The pain is neuritic in nature and radiates from a site near the metatarsal heads into the toes. At first, pain occurs only on weight bearing but ultimately occurs even at rest. *Taking the weight off the feet is not as important as removing the shoes.* This desire to remove the shoe and massage and manipulate the foot is indicative of neuralgia. Mere rest does not afford relief.

Pressure *between* the metatarsal heads reproduces the pain, whereas metatarsalgia without neoplasm causes tenderness *at* the metatarsal heads. Compression of the metatarsal heads together also causes pain in the neoplasm. Numbness and hypalgesia of the contiguous aspects of the toes may be elicited and a palpable tumor is frequently found.

Treatment is that of supporting the transverse arch in a suitable broad shoe. Local injection of steroids often gives relief, but surgical excision of the neoplasm may ultimately be required.

INTERMETATARSOPHALANGEAL BURSITIS

Inflammation of the intermetatarsophalangeal bursa can cause enlargement of the bursa, which forces traction upon the interdigital nerve causing a Morton's-neuralgia-type syndrome.

The intermetatarsophalangeal bursae lie between the heads of the second and third, third and fourth, and the fourth and fifth metatarsal bones. The bursae lie superior to the transverse metatarsal ligament,

162

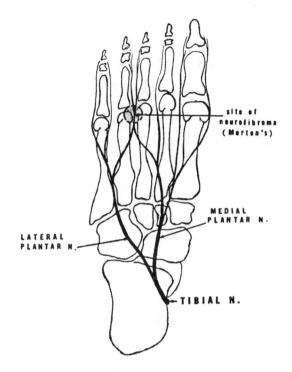

FIGURE 122. Morton's neuralgia. Morton's neuralgia results from a neurofibroma of the interdigital nerve. The most frequent site is the third branch of the medial plantar nerve as it merges with the lateral plantar nerve to form the digital nerve between the third and fourth toes. Pain occurs in the area and hypalgesia can be elicited in the opposing areas of the toes.

which in turn lies directly above the neurovascular bundle (Fig. 123, see also Fig. 51).

The pain, like that of classic Morton's neuralgia, presents as acute pain under and in between the metatarsal heads, usually the fourth digital nerve between the third and fourth metatarsals. It is described as shooting or burning, often radiating into the toes, and is made worse by walking or prolonged standing, especially when wearing tight-fitting shoes. Morton (Thomas G.) considered the condition a result of pinching of the nerve between the metatarsal heads, but as the nerves are on the plantar side of the transverse metatarsal ligament this explanation has been refuted.

Inflammation of the metatarsophalangeal joint, the transverse metatarsal ligament, or the *bursa* were therefore implicated. Traction upon the nerve rather than compression appears to be the mechanism of neuritis. As the fourth interdigital nerve is usually formed by a union of the medial and lateral plantar nerves, this terminal nerve does not yield to elongation and thus is more vulnerable. During toe extension, which occurs at each

163

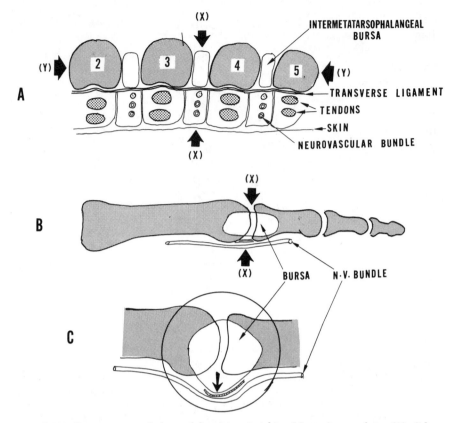

FIGURE 123. Intermetatarsophalangeal bursitis mimicking Morton's neuralgia. (A), Schematic view of intermetatarsophalangeal bursa in relationship to the transverse metatarsal ligament and the interdigital neurovascular bundle. X depicts direct digital pressure from the examiner to reproduce pain. Y shows compression of the metatarsal heads to allegedly entrap the digital nerves. (B), Lateral view of normal bursa, transverse ligament and neurovascular bundle relationship. (C), Inflamed swollen bursa elongating the neurovascular bundle causing traction upon the nerve and contiguous blood supply.

toe-off in the gait, the nerve is stretched across the transverse ligament, also compressing the accompanying blood vessels and causing an ischemic neuritis.

Diagnosis

Clinically, compression of the forefoot to approximate the metatarsal heads, or direct compression of the space in between the metatarsal heads (X and Y in Figure 123) between the fingers of the examiner reproduces the pain. Injection of an anesthetic agent in the bursal space (not neces-

164

sarily under fluoroscopy or with intra-articular dye) may confirm the diagnosis and be therapeutically beneficial.

Treatment

Injection of dye into the bursa identifies the presence and the site of the bursa. This injection, followed by infiltration through the same needle of an anesthetic and steroid suspension, frequently relieves the patient's symptoms for long periods.

Correction of faulty footwear and correction of pronation must also be instituted, as well as oral anti-inflammatory medication. Recurrence may require surgical resection of the bursa.

INTERDIGITAL NEURITIS

Other interdigital nerves may be involved and cause pain. Superficial to the transverse metatarsal ligament, the interdigital nerves pass forward from the sole of the foot to reach the dorsum of the foot. If the toes are hyperextended at the metatarsal joints, the nerves are angulated over the ligament. If there is also some abnormal pressure, a "throbbing" type of pain is felt in the involved toes. The pain persists after weight bearing and the patient tends to remove the shoe and massage the painful area.

Tenderness can be elicited by pressure *between* the metatarsal heads. This is contrary to metatarsalgia in which the pain occurs mostly during weight bearing and tenderness is elicited by pressure directly upon the metatarsal heads. If the injection of lidocaine (Novocain) between the metatarsal heads relieves the pain, the diagnosis of interdigital neuritis is confirmed.

Treatment consists of preventing hyperextension of the toes. Abnormal occupational posture, such as that depicted in Figure 124, must be corrected, and the female patient urged to avoid high-heeled shoes. A metatarsal pad or bar that flexes the toes may help. Shoes should have adequate width across the metatarsal heads and low heels. If symptoms persist, surgical release of the entrapped nerve must be considered.

POSTERIOR TIBIAL NERVE ENTRAPMENT
(TARSAL TUNNEL SYNDROME)

Pain paresthesia can occur in the plantar aspect of the foot and toes due to extrinsic or intrinsic pressure neuropathy of the posterior tibial nerve from its site of entry. The posterior tibial nerve passes under the flexor retinaculum, under the medial malleolus, to the motor or sensory terminal nerves of the medial or lateral plantar branches or posterior calcaneal

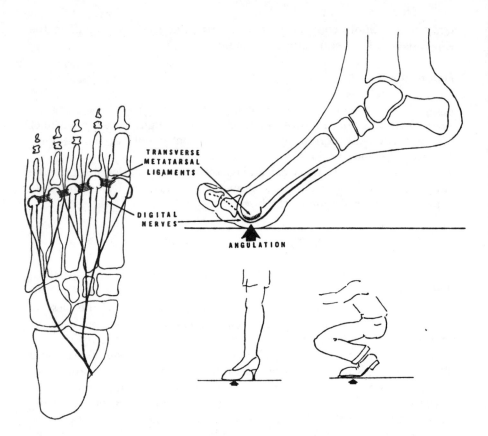

FIGURE 124. Entrapment of the interdigital nerve. The interdigital nerves are sensory to the toes. They come from the plantar nerves in the sole of the foot then pass across the transverse metatarsal ligament to the dorsum of the toes. If they are angulated at the ligament by posture and weight bearing, pain in the foot and numbness of the toes may result.

branches. The laciniate ligament forms a roof over the bony depression behind the medial malleolus converting the area into a tarsal tunnel.

Peripheral nerves, richly endowed with blood supply, have flexibility to elongate or recoil as a joint across which they extend flexes or extends. The nerve axon membrane acts as a sodium pump that requires adenosine triphosphate (ATP) to function. ATP degrades to adenosine diphosphate (ADP) which requires oxygen. If oxygen is restricted, ATP does not form and nerve conduction is impaired.

When a peripheral nerve is entrapped in its tunnel, as may be the posterior tibial nerve, the resultant edema and then ultimately scar formation inhibit the blood supply and limit the full elongation (uncoiling) of the nerve during joint movement. As the nerve elongates, if there is scarring limitation, this lengthening constricts the nerve further and compresses the intrinsic as well as extrinsic blood supply of the nerve.

As the posterior tibial nerve enters the tarsal tunnel (Fig. 125), the calcaneal branch emerges above or through the laciniate ligament to supply sensory innervation to the heel. After leaving the tunnel, the nerve passes deep to the sole of the foot and divides into a calcaneal branch and the medial and lateral plantar branches. These branches innervate the intrinsic muscles of the foot and supply the sensory branches to the sole. The medial branch carries sensation from the medial three and a half toes and the medial aspect of the sole. The lateral plantar nerve supplies the lateral half of the sole and the other outer toes.

Pressure upon the plantar branches or the posterior tibial nerve within the tunnel can occur from trauma, such as a fall with the patient landing on the feet, standing on a ladder with soft shoes, or acute pronation or acute strain upon a chronically pronated foot that causes impingement of the nerves between the tarsal bones and the sharp edge of the abductor hallucis muscle. Pressure also may occur from an ill-fitting longitudinal arch support that is too high in the arch.

The pathophysiology of nerve compression within the tunnel is initially local edema and cellular infiltrate with gradual vacuolization of the myelin sheath. This gradually leads to axon degeneration and then to Wallerian degeneration.

Diagnosis

The pain of entrapment of the posterior tibial nerve in the tarsal tunnel may be nocturnal or paresthetic ("burning") or numbness. It may be felt when standing or reclining. The distribution of the pain or numbness depends upon which nerve branch is most affected and is usually from behind the medial malleolus, over the plantar surface of the foot, the dorsum of the toes, or if the calcaneal branch is affected, the heel of the foot (see Fig. 125).

Diagnosis is made by the history of pain or numbness in the area of distribution of the plantar nerve. Tenderness can be elicited over the nerve behind the medial malleolus. A positive Tinel's sign can be elicited by tapping the nerve at the site. The dermatomal pattern can be elicited by light touch, pinprick testing, hyperesthesia, or impaired two-point discrimination. There may be motor (muscle) impairment or loss (weakness) of the toe flexors at their proximal joints. There may be atrophy of the abductor hallucis or the toe intrinsics.

Diagnostic tests may confirm the diagnosis. An electromyogram (EMG) may reveal decreased conduction across the tunnel and ultimately demyelization of the involved muscles. A local anesthetic injected into the tunnel can diagnostically (and therapeutically) decrease or eliminate the

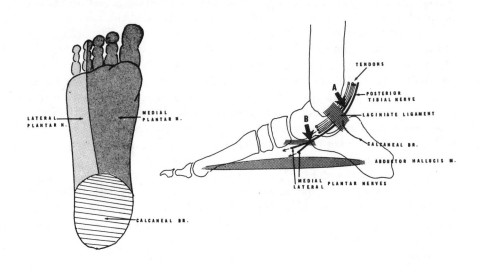

FIGURE 125. Entrapment of the posterior tibial nerve and its plantar branches. The posterior tibial nerve passes in a tunnel under the laciniate (talocalcaneal) ligament. It is accompanied by the tendons on the posterior tibial and flexor digitorum longus. The posterior tibial nerve branches into the plantar nerves and gives off a calcaneal branch. The plantar nerves supply the small muscles of the sole and their sensory distribution is shown in figure on the left.

paresthesia. Application of a tourniquet above the ankle can diagnostically reproduce the symptoms.

Treatment

When severe pronation exists and is considered to be a causative or contributing factor, every form of treating pronation should be employed. A short-leg cast or short-leg polypropylene splint to limit plantar flexion, dorsiflexion, and pronation-supination for several weeks may be beneficial. Steroids and anesthetic agents into the tarsal tunnel are of value, as is the use of oral steroids or anti-inflammatory drugs. In long existing symptomatic neuropathy, transcutaneous nerve stimulation is worth attempting. This form of treatment is of value if symptoms persist after decompression.

After a reasonable period of nonsurgical treatment with persistence of symptoms, surgical decompression is justified. This procedure is done after insuring an avascular field by Esmarch bandage or pressure dressing and pneumatic tourniquet. The retinaculum and laciniate ligament are excised, and the entire nerve is freed of constricting bands. Postoperatively, compression dressings with or without a short-leg cast or splint are employed.

Differential Diagnosis

With the assumption that the vast majority of tarsal tunnel syndromes are traumatic and mechanical, the possibility of diabetic neuropathy, rheumatoid arthritis, gout, or heavy-metal neuritis must be considered. The presence of neoplasms or ganglion is also a possibility.

<h2 style="text-align:center">ANTERIOR TIBIAL NEURITIS</h2>

Pain can be felt when the deep peroneal nerve is injured on the dorsum of the foot. This nerve (previously called the *anterior tibial* nerve) accompanies the dorsalis pedis artery and becomes superficial below the cruciate

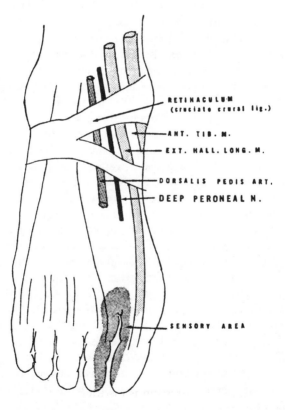

RETINACULUM
(cruciate crural lig.)

ANT. TIB. M.

EXT. HALL. LONG. M.

DORSALIS PEDIS ART.

DEEP PERONEAL N.

SENSORY AREA

FIGURE 126. Trauma to the deep peroneal nerve. The deep peroneal nerve becomes superficial as it emerges below the cruciate crural ligament. There it is vulnerable to trauma causing pain and numbness in the area shown in the diagram.

169

crural ligament. At this point, there is little tissue protecting the nerve (Fig. 126). It overlies the tarsal bones and is exposed to direct trauma. A poorly designed shoe is often the cause of trauma. Sensory involvement is at the dorsal cleft between the first and second toes. Some weakness of the big toe extensor may be elicited. There may be tenderness over the nerve which can be diagnostically relieved by an injection of lidocaine (Novocain).

REFLEX SYMPATHETIC DYSTROPHY

Reflex sympathetic dystrophy is a painful swelling of the foot, or feet, due to vasomotor instability. It has been termed Sudeck's atrophy, sympathetic reflex dystrophy, and minor causalgia. The condition in the leg and foot is similar to the minor reflex dystrophy of the shoulder-hand-finger syndrome.

The circulation of the leg and foot must be clarified, as abnormal variations are little understood. *Arterial* circulation is a combination of gravity, left ventricular cardiac impulse, and arterial tonus (Fig. 127). As the arterial blood reaches the capillaries there is tissue exchange of oxygenation with removal of metabolites. If there is an increase in arterial flow due to increased pressure or arterial relaxation, or both, there is an increase in capillary blood volume and pressure. If there is a decrease in venous and lymphatic outflow, there is an increase in capillary pressure and extracellular extravasation edema results.

Due to an increase in blood flow, arteriolar dilatation, and capillary engorgement, there is an increase in tissue temperature. The cause of increased edema due to a decrease in venous and lymphatic flow is diminution of the *pumping* action of the lower leg muscles. The major pump of the lower leg is the venous and lymphatic plexus between the gastroc-soleus muscles. Due to alternating rhythmic contraction and relaxation of the gastroc-soleus muscle group, the venous and lymphatic flow results.

The gastroc-soleus muscle group can only contract and elongate with adequate ankle plantar flexion and dorsiflexion. The action literally *squeezes* the flow in an antigravity direction. Due to one-way valves of the venous system, the venous blood is pumped upward with no distal return. As well as deficient pumping action causing edema, deficient valvular action can also result in edema. Dilatation of the veins can cause relative valvular insufficiency. Once the blood reaches the pelvic abdominal level, it must be further pumped cephalad. This pumping action exists via abdominal pressure upon the vena cava vessels, then on up to the pulmonary cardiac system. Prevention of edema therefore requires:

1. Adequate pumping action of the gastroc-soleus group.
2. Adequate ankle joint range of motion.

170

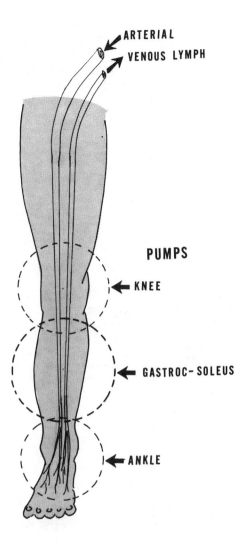

ARTERIAL

VENOUS LYMPH

PUMPS

KNEE

GASTROC-SOLEUS

ANKLE

FIGURE 127. Vascular "pumps" of the lower extremity. The venous and lymphatic return from the leg are principally the gastroc-soleus muscles with their pumping action. This muscular action requires active plantar flexion and dorsiflexion of the ankle, plus repeated flexion extension of the knee, and leg elevation.

3. Balance of arterial blood supply to venous lymphatic blood flow.
4. Efficient venous valves.
5. Periodic elimination of gravity.

In Sudeck's atrophy, one form of lymphedema, there is sympathetic vascular instability. The arteriolar muscle tone is diminished, thus causing vasodilatation. As there is excessive sympathetic venous discharge, there is also excessive perspiration and pilo erection (Fig. 128).

The mechanism by which reflex sympathetic dystrophy occurs remains conjectional but it occurs following trauma in most instances and in people who have a vasomotor instability. The condition was originally described in the Civil War following bullet injuries contiguous to nerves but

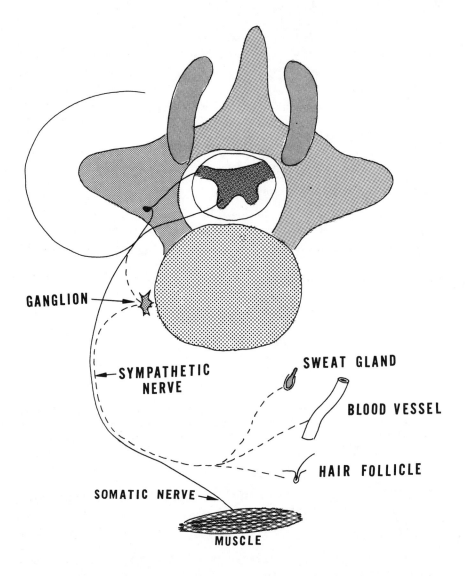

FIGURE 128. Neurologic pathway of sympathetic nervous system.

not in severance of nerves. Because the pain presented as "burning" it was originally termed *causalgia* (burning pain). The condition was one of hyperesthesia and hyperalgesia: excessive sensitivity of distal portions of extremities. Originally, it was thought to occur mostly in the upper extremity, but ultimately was similarly found in the lower extremity. Recently, reflex sympathetic dystrophy has been divided into *major* (causalgia, phantom limb, and thalamar syndrome) and *minor* (reflex sympathetic dystrophy, postmyocardial infarct, posthemiplegia, postinjection cast, and shoulder-hand-finger syndrome).

Minor reflex sympathetic dystrophy aptly termed leg-foot-toe syndrome usually begins in the foot, the distal portion of the lower extremity. Early, there may be atrophy of the hair follicles although ultimately the hair grows coarse, thick, and erect. The foot may be swollen, pale and bluish or pink in color, cold or warm, and dry although usually excessively moist. All are signs of excessive sympathetic vasomotor abnormality. Hypersensitivity is usual.

As the condition persists, there is osteoporosis of the bones of the foot with atrophic joint changes. Clinically, touch may not be tolerated and tolerance to heat or cold not accepted. Mobilization of the tarsal or metatarsal may not only be painful but limited. Anxiety has been considered to be an integral part of the syndrome. There are many who consider reflex sympathetic dystrophy to occur only in nervous, anxious patients. In fact, they believe it is caused by the vasomotor instability of anxious patients. This relationship of cause and effect remains controversial.

As the condition progresses, especially if untreated, the subcutaneous tissues atrophy and the skin becomes thin and shiny. The muscles atrophy and contract. The bones become osteoporetic and the joints undergo atrophic arthritic changes. The foot becomes free of pain but totally rigid and useless.

Treatment

Upon recognition of reflex sympathetic dystrophy, the sympathetic nervous innervation should be interrupted, and active range of motion exercises instituted, encouraged, and supervised. Chemical sympathectomy can be performed by anesthetic block of paraspinous sympathetic ganglia. Epidural injections of dilute anesthetic agents at the L_2-L_3 levels are very effective. Venous occlusion of the involved extremity by a sphygmomanometer and injection of guanethedine into the tissues distal to the cuff has been advocated. A 10 minute or more occlusion has been recommended, but too rapid or too early release of the guanethedine into the general circulation can cause disasterous hypotensive vascular complications. Propolonol, a beta-adrenergic inhibitor, has been claimed as effective as has chlorpromazine in large oral doses.

At first, resting the extremity is desirable and, in fact, may be mandatory due to the patient's reaction to pain. Frequent elevation of the entire extremity for intervals throughout the day and night is mandatory. Local application of warm moist or cold moist compresses if, and as, tolerated is beneficial. Alternating these applications, that is, hot-cold contrast baths, is claimed beneficial by some patients but are considered intolerable by others.

Active, passive, or active-assistive range of motion of the ankle in plantar flexion or dorsiflexion should be instituted early. This initiates the "pumping" action of the gastroc-soleus muscle group, delays or prevents contracture, and decreases the edema. Compression dressings by repeated elastic wrapping beginning distally and progressing proximally decreases the edema.

As soon as tolerated, the patient should be placed on heel cord stretching exercises, gastroc-resistive exercises, for stretching and walking. The statement "most cases of reflex sympathetic dystrophy will recover within two years regardless of treatment" is untrue. Atrophic joints, fibrosed muscles, and contracted ligaments and tendons *do not* revert back to normal tissues.

Reflex sympathetic dystrophy is far more frequent than medical literature would indicate and, because it results from innocuous conditions, such as sprains, strains, casted simple fractures, minor trauma, and innocuous laceration, it may not be suspected. Early recognition and early vigorous treatment are usually effective.

COMMON PERONEAL NERVE PALSY

Injury to the common peroneal nerve as it curves around the neck of the fibula will result in weakness of the evertors and dorsiflexors of the foot and cause hypalgesia on the lateral aspect of the leg and the dorsal aspect of the foot. Pain can be elicited by forcefully placing the foot into plantar flexion and inversion, which stretches the peroneal nerve. Tenderness can frequently be elicited at the fibular neck and procaine infiltration there may relieve symptoms.

REFERRED NEURITIC PAIN

The nerve roots that make up the sciatic nerve may be injured, causing neurologic signs in the foot and ankle. The most common cause of this is irritation from a herniated lumbar disk. The exact location of the disk involved is depicted in Figure 129. The dermatome deficiency indicates the nerve root involved (Fig. 130). This, in association with specific motor function (see Fig. 121) loss and reflex changes, will locate the level of spinal involvement.

174

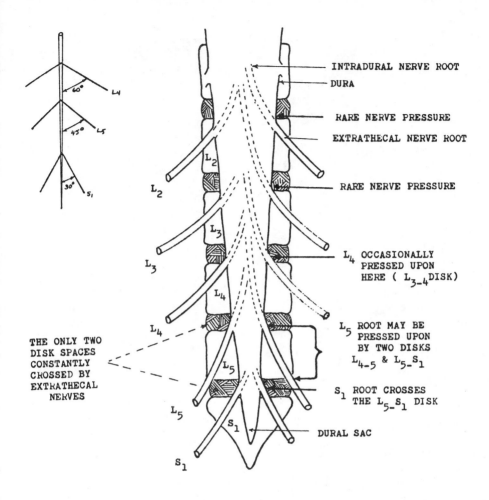

FIGURE 129. Relationship of nerve roots to disk spaces.

The diagnosis is made by a history of the pain, usually in the low back, with radiation down the posterior aspect of the leg into the calf, ankle, and even the toes. It is worse on straining. Examination finds limited low back flexibility, paraspinous spasm causing functional scoliosis, and a positive streight-leg-raising test on the involved side.

SPASTIC PARALYSIS

The foot is involved in spastic conditions resulting from upper motor neuron lesions. In the young, the cause of this is usually cerebral palsy

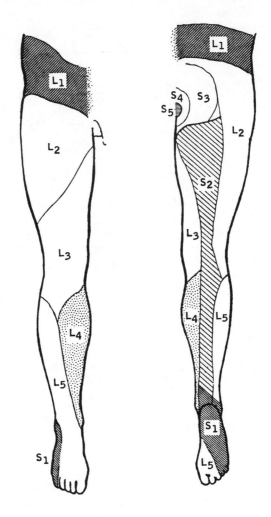

FIGURE 130. Dermatome mapping of lumbar and sacral roots.

and in the adult a cerebrovascular accident. The findings of hyperactive deep tendon reflexes, spasticity, clonus, and positive Babinski signs reveal the neurologic causes. The etiology of upper motor neuron lesions is beyond the scope of this book.

The functional abnormality of the foot in the spastic lower extremity is that of equinovarus in which the toes are unable to clear the floor during walking. Because the foot is plantar flexed the patient cannot place the heel on the ground. Treatment seeks to prevent contractures of the Achilles tendon and to strengthen the ankle dorsiflexors and evertors. The

176

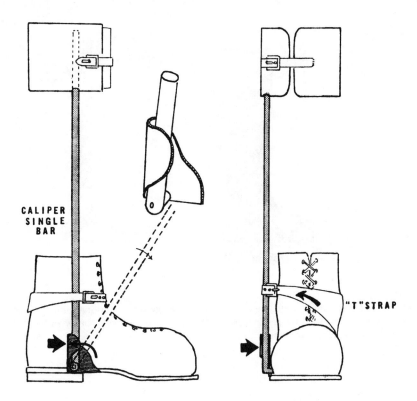

CALIPER
SINGLE
BAR

"T"STRAP

FIGURE 131. Short leg brace with right-angle stop. This short leg brace stops plantar flexion of the foot at a right angle to prevent drop foot or equinus. It may have a single or a double upright bar. The pull of the "T" strap corrects the inversion when connected to an inside bar.

Achilles tendon can be stretched by active and passive exercises often with the assistance of braces.

Bracing

Excessive plantar flexion can be prevented by the use of an ankle joint right-angle stop on a short leg caliper brace (Fig. 131), either single or double bar. A medial "T" strap can be used to pull the ankle toward the bar and thus counteract inversion of the foot. If the foot is flail or has minimal spasticity, a "piano-wire" brace may be all that is necessary to overcome the drop foot and thus permit clearance from the floor during gait (Fig. 132). A night brace may be worn to stretch the Achilles tendon by keeping the foot dorsiflexed during sleeping hours (Fig. 133). Certain types of equinovarus or those resistant to exercise and bracing may be helped surgically by Achilles tendon lengthening or by tenotomy of the

177

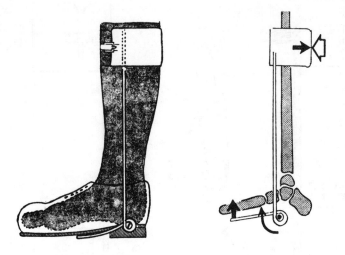

FIGURE 132. Piano-wire dorsiflexion brace. When the gastrocnemius has minimal spasticity or in a flaccid drop foot, the resilient piano wire elevates the anterior portion of the foot so it clears the floor during walking.

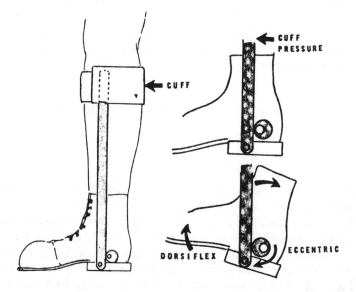

FIGURE 133. Achilles tendon stretching night brace. The eccentric ankle joint forces the bar to varying degrees altering the ankle dorsiflexion. The cuff affords counter pressure. In the right lower picture the rotation of the eccentric joint has forced the foot into dorsiflexion.

178

posterior tibial tendon and tenotomy of the flexor digitorum longus. The valgus foot that may result from these tenotomies is often preferable to the disability caused by severe equinovarus.

BIBLIOGRAPHY

BENTLEY, FH AND SCHLAPP, W: *Effects of pressure on conduction in peripheral nerve.* J Physiol (Lond) 102:72, 1943.

BETTS, LO: *Morton's metatarsalgia: Neuritis of the fourth digital nerve.* Med J Aust 1:514, 1940.

BONICA, JJ: *Causalgia and other reflex sympathetic dystrophies.* Postgrad Med 53:143, 1973.

BOSLEY, CG AND CAIRNEY, PC: *The intermetatarsophalangeal bursa—Its significance in Morton's metatarsalgia.* J Bone Joint Surg 62-B:184, 1980.

BOVILL, EG: *Diseases of nerves.* In DuVRIES, HL (ED): *Surgery of the Foot.* CV Mosby, St Louis, 1965, p 279.

CAILLIET, R: *Bracing for spasticity.* In LICHT, S (ED): *Orthotics Etcetera. Physical Medicine Library, vol 9.* Elizabeth Licht Publisher, New Haven, 1966, p 365.

CARROW, H AND McCUE, F: *Reflex sympathetic dystrophy syndrome.* Lancet 1:1226, 1976.

CULLEN, CH: *Causalgia: Diagnosis and treatment.* J Bone Joint Surg 30-B:467, 1948.

DENNY-BROWN, D AND BRENNER, C: *Paralysis of nerve induced by direct pressure and by tourniquet.* Archives of Neurology and Psychiatry 51:1, 1944.

DENNY-BROWN, D AND DOHERTY, MM: *Effects of transient stretching of peripheral nerves.* Archives of Neurology and Psychiatry 54:116, 1945.

EDWARDS, WG, ET AL: *The tarsal tunnel syndrome: Diagnosis and treatment.* JAMA 207:716, 1969.

FRAZIER, FW: *Persistent post-sympathetic pain treated by connective tissue massage.* Physiotherapy 64:211, 1978.

GILLIAT, RW AND WILSON, TG: *A pneumatic tourniquet test in the carpal tunnel syndrome.* Lancet 11:595, 1953.

GOODGOLD, J, KOPELL, HP, AND SPIELHOLZ, NI: *The tarsal-tunnel syndrome. Objective diagnostic criteria.* N Engl J Med 273:742, 1965.

HANNINGTON-KIFF, JG: *Intravenous regional sympathetic block with guanethedine.* Lancet 1:1019, 1974.

HAYMAKER, W AND WOODHALL, B: *Peripheral Nerve Injuries: Principles of Diagnosis,* ed 2. WB Saunders, Philadelphia, 1959.

HERTZLER, AE: *Bursitides of the plantar surface of the foot.* Am J Surg 1:117, 1926.

JOHNSON, EW AND ORTIZ, PR: *Electrodiagnosis of tarsal tunnel syndrome.* Archives of Physical Medicine 47:776, 1966.

KOPELL, HP AND THOMPSON, WAL: *Peripheral Entrapment Neuropathies.* Williams & Wilkins, Baltimore, 1963, p 171.

KOZIN, F, ET AL: *Reflex sympathetic dystrophy syndrome. I. Clinical and histological studies: Evidence for bilaterality, response to corticosteroids and articular involvement.* Am J Med 60:321, 1976.

LAM, SJS: *A tarsal-tunnel syndrome.* Lancet 2:1354, 1962.

MARINACCI, AA: *Clinical Electromyography.* San Lucas Press, Los Angeles, 1955.

MORTON, TG: *A peculiar and painful affection of the fourth metatarsophalangeal articulation.* Am J Med Sci 71:37, 1876.

OESTER, YT AND MAYER, JH: *Motor Examination of Peripheral Nerve Injuries.* Charles C Thomas, Springfield, Ill, 1960.

OMER, G AND THOMAS, S: *Treatment of causalgia: Review of cases at Brooke General Hospital.* Tex Med 67:93, 1971.

PERRY, J: *Orthopedic management of the lower extremity in the hemiplegic patient.* Journal of American Physical Therapists Association 46:345, 1966.

STAMP, W: *Bracing in cerebral palsy.* J Bone Joint Surg 44-A:1457, 1962.

TOUMEY, JW: *Occurrence and management of reflex sympathetic dystrophy (causalgia of the extremities).* J Bone Joint Surg 30-A:883, 1948.

CHAPTER 12

The Foot in Diabetes

As the population median age increases, so also does the incidence of diabetes and its complications due to vascular changes, which manifest in the foot. As many as one in six diabetic patients may have a foot abnormality. Ischemia of the foot is very rare under the age of 40, but in the diabetic patient, impairment is classically in the popliteal, tibial, and foot blood vessels. The greatest complication of diabetes is vascular changes that lead to peripheral gangrene and diabetic peripheral neuropathy.

No foot problem in the diabetic patient can be taken lightly. Surgical excision of a callus is a major procedure and the ingrown toenail is a serious lesion. In diabetes, the foot with impaired circulation is susceptible to gangrenous changes and infection. Proper toenail care is mandatory, as is the need for properly fitting shoes and foot cleanliness with proper drying.

Diabetes mellitus causes two forms of vascular disease, large-vessel disease and small-vessel disease. Even though both are vascular they cause distinctive syndromes.

LARGE-VESSEL DISEASE

This condition is essentially one of arteriosclerosis with internal plaque formation forming thrombi and luminal narrowing. One symptom may be intermittent claudication, in which painful cramping of the leg occurs during ambulation and ceases after a period of rest. The pain is usually diffusely in the calf muscle.

Clinical examination of the leg reveals diminished or absent pulsation of the dorsalis pedis artery or the posterior tibial artery. The skin color is usually blanched with increased blanching on elevation of the leg and then demonstrates rubor in dependency. The skin may appear thin and the hair on the dorsum of the toes sparce or absent. There is a deficient venous filling time. Venous filling time is determined by elevating the leg for two minutes then placing it in a dependent position and measuring the time for venous filling. If it takes longer than 20 seconds, the venous filling time is considered delayed and arterial supply by large vessels is considered to exist.

SMALL-VESSEL DISEASE

This is entirely different from large-vessel disease and is frequently accompanied by neuropathy. Fat plaques do not form in the intima or project into the lumen. In small-vessel disease, there is thickening and formation of amorphous tissue within the basement membrane of the vessels. It is this thickening that produces the mechanical barrier and occurs in the tiny arterioles and capillaries. In small-vessel disease, there are venous changes (in the vessels) causing black patches in the skin of the foot, due to subcutaneous hemorrhaging.

DIABETIC NEUROPATHY

This neuropathy is a complication of small-vessel disease of the vasa nervorum. A distinct sequence of events occurs with early diminished skin sensation (hypalgesia and hypesthesia). The deep tendon reflexes become diminuted. In the performance of electromyography (EMG), nerve conduction testing, there is a delay on motor and sensory nerve conduction due to segmental demyelination. As the vasa nervorum changes occur, there is also progressive drying and scaling (anhidrosis). Proprioception becomes impaired and a Charcot joint may result.

Due to impaired sensation, trauma to the foot may occur without patient awareness until the injury is deep and serious. Vibration sense is lost early whereas touch and position sense is frequently retained.

TREATMENT

Treatment of the lower extremity in diabetic patients is both nonsurgical and surgical.

Nonsurgical

From the onset of diabetes, the patient must constantly be made aware of potential damage and the need for proper care of the feet. Patient education and constant periodic examination are mandatory and ongoing. Trauma to the foot must be avoided with proper foot wear. The patient should never wear shoes without socks. Socks should be washed until they can shrink no more. Properly fitting socks are neither too large nor too small. If too large, socks will wrinkle; if too small they will cause constriction. They must also be soft, warm, and undarned.

Proper foot care requires daily washing with soap and lukewarm or cool water, meticulous drying by blotting rather than rubbing (taking particular care with the spaces between the toes), and then massaged with a lanolin cream to soften the skin. The toenails should be cut straight across to prevent ingrowing of the edges. If this is difficult for the patient, it should be done by a podiatrist or a trained relative. Older patients should have periods of rest during the day with the shoes removed.

Edema must be evaluated, avoided, and if present be treated vigorously. Frequent leg elevation during the day is beneficial. However, elevation of the legs too high or for too long should be avoided in the presence of arterial insufficiency regardless of the extent of edema. Carefully fitted elastic hose of total leg length are beneficial. Exercises that also help include elevation of the leg, plantar flexion and dorsiflexion of the ankle, inversion and eversion of the foot, and plantar flexion (curling) and dorsiflexion (extension) of the toes.

Heat applied directly to the feet must be carefully avoided. Because of impaired skin sensation, trauma may occur and ulcerations may exist unnoticed by the patient until the injury is deep and serious. Secondary infection and distal gangrene result frequently. Because half of the diabetic patients who develop ulcers and gangrene eventually require amputation, it is imperative that preventive measures be instituted early and energetically. Reflex heating by applying heating pads to the lower abdomen or upper thighs is the only safe application of heat. Wool socks may be worn to bed but electric pads and hot-water bottles should be avoided.

Daily exercises of the feet and legs must be initiated and performed daily. Exercises consist of gentle heel cord stretching and gastroc-soleus standing and sitting exercises. Alternate elevation and dependency of the leg should be performed frequently during the day, both with the shoes on and barefoot. Exercise is the best vasodilator available to the patient. Intermittent walking to the point of pain and *slightly further,* followed by standing and sitting, with a avoidance of excessive periods of standing or sitting, should be done daily. Avoidance of restrictive garments, such as garters and tight mid-lower-leg stockings is mandatory.

Meticulous *early* care of any open wound must be stressed. An antibacterial soap (liquid hexochlorophine) in a cool solution should be used. Any dead or damaged tissue must be carefully removed by a surgeon or qualified podiatrist. Hydrogen peroxide may be used to debride the damaged area. Local antibiotics are rarely of value, in fact, strong disinfectants, ointments, and chemical compounds are best avoided.

Surgical

Lumbar sympathectomy can theoretically enhance the development of collateral blood supply. However, it is of no value in small-vessel disease as the vessels involved have no muscle coat, hence, no possible vasodilation. Lumbar sympathectomies also are considered of little value as many diabetic patients have already had autosympathectomy as a result of their neuropathy. Lumbar sympathectomies have exponents, but only in the presence of large-vessel disease. Sympathectomy, if considered valuable in large-vessel disease, can be performed by paraspinous chemical sympathectomy or epidural chemical sympathectomy followed by surgical sympathectomy.

Endarterectomy preceded by diagnostic arteriography has recently become clarified and beneficial. Vascular surgery recently has made vast strides and can benefit the diabetic patient before the serious complications occur.

Amputations require careful evaluation of the exact level of amputation. So-called "dry" gangrene, is a sequala of small-vessel occlusion with specific localization and self-amputation (autoamputation). "Wet" gangrene implies occlusion of the venous portion (venule) of the circulation, and stasis occurs causing edema. Moist tissue is usually infected. Wet gangrene requires careful decision of the level of elective amputation, dependent upon the state of circulation and the ultimate rehabilitation of function with or without orthotics.

Only if the patient is thoroughly educated and follows a closely supervised and regimented program is there a chance to walk on two good feet in later years.

BIBLIOGRAPHY

COLLENS, WS, ET AL: *Conservative management of gangrene in diabetic patients.* JAMA 181:692, 1962.

CONRAD, MC: *Large and small artery occlusion in diabetics and nondiabetics with severe vascular disease.* Circulation 30:83, 1967.

DETAKETS, G: *Diabetic vascular disease.* Southern Med J 57:1143, 1964.

ELLENBERG, M: *Diabetic neuropathy: Clinical aspects.* Metabolism 25:1627, 1979.

FABERBERG, SE: *Diabetic neuropathy—A clinical and histological study on the significance of avascular affectation.* Acta Med Scand (Suppl) 345:164, 1959.

GOLDENBERG, S, ET AL: *Nonatheromatous peripheral vascular disease of the lower extremities in diabetes mellitus.* Diabetes 8:261, 1959.

PEDERSEN, J AND OLSEN, S: *Small-vessel disease of the lower extremity in diabetes mellitus.* Acta Med Scand 171:551, 1962.

WHITEHOUSE, FC AND BLOCK, MA: *The problems of the diabetic foot.* J Am Geriat Soc 12:1043, 1964.

CHAPTER 13

Dermatologic Conditions
of the Foot

There are a number of painful dermatologic conditions of the foot, which include plantar warts, calluses, corns, and various forms of "dermatitis." These are all capable of interfering with normal foot mobility and gait.

CALLUS

A callus is a thickening of the skin, either diffuse or circumscribed, in an area exposed to persistent abnormal pressure or friction. Abnormal foot mechanics precede their formation. In conditions in which the transverse arches are depressed, weight bearing by the metatarsal heads will lead to the formation of plantar calluses. In the markedly inverted foot, pressure upon the fifth metatarsal head will result in a callus there. If the toes are clawed or hammered, the skin over the protruding interphalangeal joints will develop calluses where it presses against the shoe.

Calluses may be confused with warts but when pared show normal papillary lines running through the hyperkeratotic area. The lines do not deviate. There may be a translucent core that is well demarcated, but there are no blood vessels in the core.

Treatment consists of application of 40 percent salicyclic acid plaster and a felt pad with the center cut out to prevent further pressure or friction. Ultimate treatment for calluses requires avoidance of the abnormal contact points by the wearing of corrective shoes. Unless the cause of abnormal foot mechanics and the sites of abnormal pressure and friction are discovered and corrected the lesion will recur after treatment.

NEUROVASCULAR CORN

A variant of corns, the neurovascular corn, may pose a diagnostic problem. It appears over a bony prominence and is sharply demarcated.

185

When pared a small blood vessel appears that lies *parallel* to the surface and not vertical as in the case of warts. The neurovascular corn can be very tender and painful. It is best treated by paring followed by the weekly application of 50 to 100 percent solution of silver nitrate. In between these treatments a 40 percent salicylic acid plaster is applied.

"SOFT" CORN

A "soft" corn is a hyperkeratotic lesion found *between* the toes. These corns usually occur between the fourth and fifth toes and are most frequently situated in the web. They result from the pressure of opposing toes and occur in a region that is constantly moist, which denys them the chance to become cornified. They are best treated by application of 40 percent salicylic acid plasters and separation of the toes by sponge rubber pads or lamb's wool. Surgical excision is often necessary, and should there be an underlying bone spur promoting corn formation, it too should be surgically removed.

PLANTAR WARTS

Plantar warts differ from calluses and are not necessarily found over bony prominences. They are sharply circumscribed with their edges clearly demarcated from the surrounding skin (Fig. 134). Their center is darker than the surrounding skin and they may have a mosaic appearance. If the surrounding skin is stretched from the "core," a small cleft appears between it and the surrounding skin. Warts are usually tender to squeezing, whereas in calluses the tenderness is usually in the bony prominences under it.

Plantar warts are simple papillomas considered to be caused by a virus. There are three varieties of plantar warts. The first is the *single* wart that often appears under a bony prominence and may, at first, be difficult to differentiate from a callus. When the wart is pared the distinct margin becomes apparent, and its surface is *dotted by small capillary tips*. The second variety is the *"mother-daughter"* type in which a large wart is surrounded by several smaller "satellite" warts. The satellite warts have the same characteristics as the center wart but in the early stages may be more vesicular than the keratotic mother. They are usually extremely painful. The third type, the *mosaic*, appears as granular calluses that are grouped in a mosaic pattern that may extend over the entire metatarsal surface. The individual cores of the mosaic resemble the single wart.

Treatments are numerous. *Surgery is contraindicated for all plantar warts* as the resulting scar may be more painful than the wart, and new warts can grow in and along the scar. The objective in treating plantar warts is always to eradicate it with the minimal amount of scarring as the

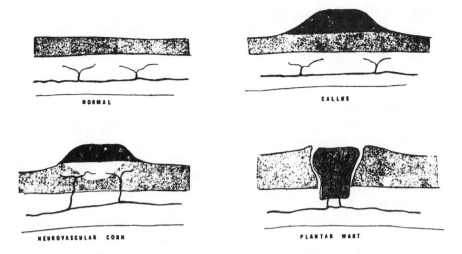

FIGURE 134. Dermatologic conditions of the foot. The *callus* is merely a hyperkeratotic area that forms at the point of persistent pressure or friction. The *neurovascular corn* is a hyperkeratotic area with an avascular translucent base that may have a blood vessel lying parallel to the surface. The *plantar wart* is a papilloma, cone shaped, with a cleft between it and the surrounding skin. Blood vessels in the *wart* are vertical and the ends are visible when pared.

scar may be as painful and disabling as the wart. Application of salicylic acid tape directly to the wart, removed and reapplied several times daily, frequently relieves symptoms in a few days and causes disappearance of the wart in several weeks. They may be curetted and the exposed base cauterized by commercial dry ice, solid carbon dioxide, or liquid nitrogen. Electrocautery may be lightly applied to the base. Plantar warts respond to radiotherpy, but great care must be exercised to protect the surrounding skin with a lead shield.

The mosaic warts may be treated by paring to the point of bleeding, then applying 100 percent silver nitrate to the capillary tips followed by swabbing with a saturated solution of trichloroacetic acid. This is followed by the application of 40 percent salicylic acid plaster held in place by moleskin for a period of one week. This procedure is repeated weekly until normal skin tissue replaces the wart.

HYPERHIDROSIS

Hyperhidrosis (excessive perspiration) may be troublesome. It creates or continues and adversely affects dermatologic conditions that must be specifically treated. In the absence of specific dermatitis, hyperhidrosis can be treated by application of 25 percent aluminum chloride solution three to four nights each week. There are many commercial antiperspirants on the market that decrease hyperhidrosis, but care must be taken that they do not cause skin sensitivity or irritation.

KERATODERMIA PLANTARIS

The entire sole around the margin of the heel may undergo diffuse thickening in which painful fissures may develop. This condition is called keratodermia plantaris and has variable causes. It may be a form of psoriasis, may be familial, or may be a nonspecific condition noted during various climatic changes. Treatment consists of softening the heel by warm foot soaks followed by massage with a lanolin salve. If the cornified layer is thick, it should be removed with a pumice stone or an emery board. Deep fissures may be treated by applying silver nitrate to them, which is momentarily painful but hastens healing. Antibiotics that are not prone to create a sensitive local absorption may be used when the fissures are infected.

ATHLETE'S FOOT

Athlete's foot is a fungus infection characterized by itchy, scaly lesions between the toes that frequently lead to fissure formation. Secondary infections are not uncommon. Prophylaxis by use of good foot hygiene is the preferred treatment, but once the foot is infected specific medications can be effectively applied.

SOFT TISSUE TUMORS

Tumors of soft tissues are rare and most often are tumors of tendon sheaths called ganglia. Being of tendon sheath origin, they are rarely malignant and require excision only when they interfere with function or comfort. Nodules may appear in the plantar fascia in the arch of the foot that are the equivalent of Dupuytren's contracture in the palm. These nodules are removed when they impair normal gait and should be biopsied to differentiate them from fibrosarcoma.

DIABETIC DERMATOLOGIC COMPLICATIONS

When dealing with dermatologic conditions of the foot, the possibility of underlying diabetes must always be considered. The tissues of diabetic patients heal poorly and the vascular impairment often associated with diabetes causes ischemia and neuropathy. Proper foot hygiene in diabetes is imperative. This has been discussed in detail in Chapter 12, The Foot in Diabetes.

BIBLIOGRAPHY

DeTakats, G: *Diabetic vascular disease.* South Med J 57:1143, 1964.

Giannestras, NJ: *Plantar keratosis, treatment by metatarsal shortening.* J Bone Joint Surg 48A:727, 1966.

Lewin, P: *The Foot and Ankle,* ed 4. Lea & Febiger, Philadelphia, 1959.

Montgomery, RM: *Dermatological care of the painful foot.* J Bone Joint Surg 46A:1129, 1964.

Whitehouse, FW and Block, MA: *The problem of the diabetic foot.* J Am Geriatr Soc 12:1045, 1964.

Index

A *t* indicates a table.
An italic number indicates a figure.

193

197

198